Questions and Answers about Vegetarians and Health

James C. Tibbetts, STL, MA

ISBN: 978-1-329-16911-1

The Scripture citations are taken in part or whole from various bibles including: *The New American Bible* (Thomas Nelson Publisher, 1970); *The Jerusalem Bible* (Doubleday & Co., 1966); *Revised Standard Version, Holy Bible from the Ancient Eastern Text*, translation from the *Aramaic of the Peshitta* by George M. Lamsa, (Harper San Francisco,1961).

Jim Tibbetts
P.O. Box 2533
Glenville, NY 12325

www.jimtibbetts.com

Library of Congress Cataloging-in-Publication Data
James C. Tibbetts
   Includes bibliographical references.

Your ISBN: 978-1-329-16911-1

Introduction

This book is a question and answer approach on plant based diets. It comes from my other books which were years of reading, collecting and researching the data about plant-based diets and fasting. My writings primarily fall into two categories:

First, the I have been looking into the diets of Jesus and Mary since the 1980's and printed the books: *Biblical Fasting* (1998); *Biblical Nutrition the Kosher Vegetarianism of Jesus and Judaism* (2003); *Biblical Nutrition Forty Days of Meditations* (2004); *Biblical Nutrition & Fasting* (2008) and *Jesus and Mary were Kosher Vegetarians, the Evidence from the Bible, the Early Church and Nutrition* (2014).

These books are foundational works which propose that Jesus and Mary were the new Adam and Eve who fasted and ate a plant-based diet, like the diet of the first Adam and Eve in the Garden of Eden (Gen. 1.29). This type of Living Foods diet or raw vegan diet is a purifying diet, it purifies the body and helps it to heal and be restored. It is beyond a simple plant-based diet, which is where most start.

I have been a vegetarian since my last two years of college 1974-1976, into fasting since about 1978 and have been into raw, living foods since the spring of 2001. I have done over 40 long fast: 7-10 days; 14; 21; 33 and 2 of 40 day juice fasts. Life is a journey and this has been part of my journey. I hope that I can share some of my experience and research in this book on Question and Answers. My other books go into these and other aspects of nutrition and fasting.

The prophet Hosea said to the kingdom of Judah, "My people are destroyed from lack of knowledge." Hos 4:6 This quote is being fulfilled today in the area of nutrition because people are being destroyed because of a lack of knowledge of how and what to eat in their dietary lifestyle and when and how to fast. In this day and age a Live-food or raw vegan diet and fasting are needed because of all the poisons, toxins, pesticides, heavy metals and other chemicals in our environment which get into our bodies. Fasting and sometimes a raw food diet can flush these out before they start to multiply and cause degenerative disease and death. My other books go into this scientific process.

May God bless your efforts as you grow in your attempt to honor the body, the Temple of the Holy Spirit. "My dear friend, I hope you are in good health and may you thrive in all other ways as you do in the spirit." 3 John 2

Sincerely in Christ

James C. Tibbetts

Question and Answers

These are general questions for the public, in a few place are journal studies citied but for the most part they are left out and can be found in Jim Tibbetts books. These are just a few of the many questions that could be asked, but they cover a lot of topics on plant-based diets.

The questions are meant to be general questions and answers and are not meant to be scholarly answers with lots of footnotes, most of them come from my writings in which I have academic citations with footnotes, but that takes away from a simple question and answer format. Hopefully this will be a benefit to many interested in this field. Peace.

The various three letter abbreviations such as Veg. are used here for ease of use and for changes and website usage.

Vegetarian Diets
(Veg. means vegetarian question)

1. Question #Veg.1 What is a vegetarian diet?

The term "vegetarian" does not mean vegetable eater but it stems from the Latin *vegetus*, which means "whole, sound, fresh, and lively, or to enliven". Most vegetarians believe that plant foods are life giving, alive and bring health. The word "diet" comes from the Greek work *dieta*, which means "way of life." A diet needs to be a lifestyle in order to be effective. And the lifestyle needs to come from the heart to be spiritual, real and true. The emphasis is on live or living foods.

"It is my view that the vegetarian manner of living, by its purely physical effect on the human temperament, would most beneficially influence the lot of mankind." Albert Einstein

In the beginning in the Garden of Eden Adam and Eve were

raw vegetarians: "God said, 'See, I give you all the seed-bearing plants that are upon the whole earth, and all the trees with seed-bearing fruit; this shall be your food." Gn 1.29

2. Question #Veg.2 What are some of the categories of vegetarians?

1. The vegans, which excludes all types of meat, poultry, fish, eggs, cheese, etc.
2. The ovo-lacto vegetarian diet which allows eggs, dairy and cheese products.
3. The lacto vegetarian diet which allows dairy products.
4. The ovo vegetarian diet which allows eggs but no dairy.
5. Raw vegetarian diet which involves all kinds of fruits and vegetables only raw and little to nothing cooked.
6. And there are many cultural movements that are partially or totally vegetarian such as Macrobiotics.

These traditional distinctions on vegetarianism are not really that helpful or necessary and only cloud the issue. Most vegetarians bounce back and forth between one and the other diet regime. And the problem is that they are really trying to define vegetarian in its relation to meat. But the real definition of the term vegetarian is based on life and vitality and wholeness and that comes from a vegetarian diet.

The SAD diets which includes the USDA's pyramid diet, are the unhealthiest diets according to the research over the last twenty years. The Health Food diets and Vegetarian diets are much healthier than the different SAD diets. The research is fairly clear of the superiority of the vegetarian diet over the meat eating diet.

3. Question #Veg.3. How does cooking relate to vegetarian diets?

Animal protein deteriorates in heating and cooking. When animal protein is heated to 212 degrees, or over 120. It deteriorates into polyscraides which are carcinagines, and then too much animal protein residue also feeds cancer cells.

The categories that are the superior diets and foods are those foods that are still living. Cooking kills the foods.

I. Living Food Diets (Superior Health)
The Raw Veggie Diets are 0% to 20% cooked
The Vegan Diets are about 10% to 30% cooked
II. Health Food Diets (Semi-healthy)
The Vegetarian Diets are about 30 to60% cooked
The Partial Vegetarian Diet are about 50 to 70% cooked
III. Standard American Diets (Unhealthy)
The Food Pyramid Diets are about 40 to 90% cooked
The Standard American Diet are about 50 to100% cooked

The reason I, first says, Health Food Diets is that these diets are "healthy" in the short term but in the long run, more than several decades on the diet they can and usually do become Semi-healthy. This is because of the cooking and commercially prepared foods and strong use of grains that can be influential in degenerative diseases. Also a healthy diet really needs to be under 80% cooked whereas the partial vegetarian and vegetarian diets usually have a lot of cooking.

The direction is obvious to go from the SAD diet to the vegetarian diet to the raw vegetarian diet. The partial or semi-vegetarian diet is only meant to be a transitional phase and one should not settle down there. Poultry is just as bad, in some cases worst then red meat.

Dr. Neal Bernard writes: "In their search for the smoking gun linking meat to cancer, scientists have discovered cancer-causing chemicals, called heterocyclicamines that form as meat is cooked. And the issue does not stop as red meat. While these carcinogens are often present in well-done beef, they have turned up in far higher levels in grilled chicken, as well as in fish." (*Cancer Research Journal*)

Cooking, baking roasting, broiling, boiling and steaming destroy from 30% to 90% of the nutrition in the food, resulting in a nutrient-deficient diet, the main cause of degenerative diseases. 97-100% of the enzymes are destroyed in cooking. Minerals are leached into the cooking water when cooking; and liquids (broth) are often poured out.

Cooked foods become so devitalized they take more energy to digest than they give and are difficult to digest.

Cooked foods shorten our life span.

Cooked foods cause far more build-up of toxins, a factor suppressing the immune system and making the body more susceptible to disease of all kinds.

Cooked foods encourage over eating, resulting in weight gain. Since they are nutrient-deficient, they leave the system still hungering for and craving food.

The natural fiber is broken down, increasing transit time of food through the gastrointestinal tract. Increased transit time means sugars ferment, proteins putrefy, and fats turn rancid, loosening toxins for absorption.

The carcinogenic substances are formed from foods-cooked or grilled over charcoal forms during some cooking procedures. The meat drippings drop onto the charcoal and carcinogenic substances are transmitted by steam onto the cooked meats.

Leucocytosis (an increase in white blood cell count and associated with a pathological condition) increases upon ingestion of cooked food.

There is poor mastication resulting in decreased saliva and enzyme flow; food is, therefore, poorly prepared for digestion.

Cooked food is most often fragmented/refined/deficient.

Cooked food is most often highly chemicalized.

Cooked food is prepared in utensils that give off toxic metal/plastic/paint particles.

Cooked food is most often addicting and promotes

4

overeating.

Finally cooked foods falsely satisfy the taste and appetite but cause abnormal cravings for sugary foods (candy, cakes, pies, ice creams, cookies, etc.) Heavy meats, richly-seasoned starches, such as breads with spreads, deep fat-fried potato and corn chips, French fries, spicy, rich grain and legume dishes also cause abnormal cravings. After such a meal, the coffee drinker craves coffee for the caffeine fix, which over-stimulates the pancreas to produce more enzymes to digest all the heavy food.

When certain foods are roasted or baked, they turn brown or golden and their taste and aroma are enhanced. This is from the Maillard reaction, which occurs when amino acids are cooked in the presence of carbohydrates (particularly reducing sugars such as glucose). This reaction can produce compounds called advanced glycocxidation endproducts (AGEs), which are of significant concern. This negative or bad effect on a macro-molecular level can be the cause of degenerative diseases in the future.

AGEs are linked to cancer and 'enhanced cancer progression,' (Ann. NY Acad. Sci.) diabetes, kidney disease, aging, (J. Am Diet. Assoc.) and neurodegenerative diseases such as Alzheimer's. (Med. Hypotheses) AGEs are also implicated in slower healing of wounds in diabetics (Diabetes) as well as diabetes-related autoimmunity. (Smith, Genetic Roulette) AGEs may reduce nutritive value, (Am. Acid) as well as increase protein stability, and therefore allergenicity. Higher levels of AGEs are also detected in patients with Creuzfeld-Jacob Disease (CJD), but it is not clear if they contribute to the disease.

This browning effect is what happens to cooked meats all the time!

Also the higher the temperature and the longer you cook meats the more they become denatured. Proteins start to become denatured over 150 degrees, that is why pasteurization tries to stay under 150 degrees. One study showed that when you fry two eggs about 50% of the protein is destroyed and you're only getting the amount of protein from one egg. Protein goes through a change when it is cooked. Protein is destroyed at 150 degrees. At this temperature the chemical body and structure of protein is 'de-natured,' and once this happens, there is nothing we can do to 'un-de-nature' protein.

One raw food expert, Malkamus said, "Protein is denatured when cooked, amino acids fuse together, making the protein unusable and when cooked, amino acids are destroyed or converted to forms that are either extremely difficult or impossible to digest." The obvious problem is that if some of the protein is destroyed by the cooking process then more protein is needed to get the minimum daily requirements.

4. Question #Veg.4   What are the food categories for raw vegan diets?

For a Raw Living Foods Diet these five categories are usually considered base foods:
1. Vegetables (green and leafy vegetables, potatoes, etc.)
2. Grains sprouted (rice, barley, millet, wheat, bulgur, etc.)
3. Legumes (beans and peas of all sorts)
4. Fruits (apples, oranges, plums, etc.)
5. Nuts and Seeds (almonds, walnuts, peanuts, etc.)

Because of its importance let me repeat this statement. The term "vegetarian" does not mean vegetable eater but it stems from the Latin *vegetus*, which means "whole, sound, fresh, and lively, or to enliven". Most vegetarians believe that plant foods are life giving, alive and bring health.

On grocery shelves, there sit more than 5,000 items processed from whole natural foods into empty edibles. Some 65% of the American adults and 25% of children under 17 now live with chronic disease which can be fed by cooked foods and commercially prepared foods. Supermarkets are places where some aisles are like funeral homes and many foods are dead foods that lie in state, laid out for the public to see!

5. Question #Veg.5 What are protein values of carnivores vs. vegans

A survey by the U.S. Dept. of Agriculture and a study in the American Journal of Clinical Nutrition shows that the vegans are the most efficient in terms of nutrition because they can consume less and get enough nutrients at the same time. They are eating more fruits and vegetables with almost double the fiber of the lactovegetarians. And their average protein intake is 35 grams, while the average American usually consumes over 100 grams.

	Meat-eaters	Lactovegetarians	Vegans
protein	85 g	55 g	35 g
fiber	4.5 g	8 g	15 g
salt	2.5 g	1.2 g	0.25 g
calories	2000 cals	1800 cals	1600 cals

Vilcabamba inhabitants in Ecuador show the largest number of centenarians of any place in the world - 1098 for every 100,000 people! According to Dr. Alexander Leaf, M.D., their average protein intake is 35-38 grams a day, and the total caloric intake is only 1200 to 1360 a day. They are almost 100 percent vegetarians."

A study in the Journal of Laboratory and Clinical Medicine showed that: "Under normal circumstances 30 to 35 grams is enough for men and some sources say 25."

A Dr. Russell Chittenden of Yale University did a protein study and concluded "that one is able to maintain good health by consuming 36 g. of protein and 2000 calories of energy daily." His conclusions were done before any dietary

7

standard was set in the U.S. "According to the report of the World Health Organization, (c. 1978) the requirements of protein for the average adult is 0.59 grams per kilogram of body weight per day. If one person weighs about 130 lbs. He must take 36 g. of protein per day."

An adult may manufacture upwards of 200 grams of protein a day but about 80% may be recycled, the amino acids are reassembled. About 20% may be lost and thus a new supply is needed from dietary intake. Thus 20% of about 200 grams is about 40 grams a day that is needed. (Nutrition in Spaceflight)

"Protein in human mother's milk (as percentage of total calories): is 5 percent." The World Health Organization's protein requirements parallel this fact. Human minimum protein requirement (according to the World Health Organization): is 5 percent of total calories. The U.S. Recommended Dietary Allowance for adult protein intake: is 10 percent of total calories." Obviously there is a big difference here, the U.S. Recommended Dietary Allowance is double what the World Health Organization states.

In a study on "Protein in the U.S. Diet," by The Journal of the American Dietetic Association, pointed out: "The levels of protein consumption in the Western nations are not nearly 'higher than enough,' they are far higher than are safe. The average American is probably getting from two to three times as much protein as he actually needs."

The average man in the U.S. eats 175% more protein than the recommended daily allowance (RDA) and the average woman eats 144% more! Surgeon General's Report on Nutrition and Health

These data suggest that during adult life, a reduction in dietary intake of fat and proteins of animal origin may contribute to a substantial reduction in the incidence of breast cancer...in population subgroups with high intake of animal

8

products. Journal of National Cancer Institute

A report from the National Academy of Sciences states: "Evidences from both epidemiological and laboratory studies suggests that high protein intake may be associated with an increased risk of cancers at certain sites." Committee on Diet, Nutrition, and Cancer of the National Research Council

Some studies in the Journal of American Dietetic, point out that 30 grams is quite adequate, and other studies have even indicated that under 10 grams might be sufficient in certain cases. (Proteins in Human Nutrition)

Allan Cott, M.D. comments in Fasting as a Way of Life that: "Controlled experiments have shown the average person can function perfectly well with protein intakes of only 30 to 35 grams per day...Studies by Dr. John W. Berg and others at the National Cancer Institute link colon cancer with high consumption of beef. ... Corroborating studies involving 112 vegetarian and 88 non-vegetarian adults, adolescents, and pregnant women reported in the Journal of Clinical Nutrition as follows:

1. The average intake of nutrients of all groups exceed those recommended by the National Research Council, with the exception of adolescent 'pure' vegetarians.
2. Nonvegetarian adolescents consume more protein, but there is no evidence that an ovo-lacto vegetarian diet failed to provide adequate diet for them or for expectant mothers.
3. There were no significant differences in height, weight, and blood pressure among the groups, but 'pure' vegetarians weighed an average of 20 pounds less.
4. Cholesterol was higher in the nonvegetarian groups. The 'pure' vegetarian diet, whatever its shortcomings, is cholesterol-free."

There's perhaps less than five cases of protein deficiency reported in the U.S. and there is over 50 million cases of protein excess in the U.S., which increases the amount and intensity of degenerative diseases.

All the above studies were concerning protein ranges of vegan (35 g.) to lacto-ovo-vegetarian (55g.) grams. Victoras Kulvinskas cited a study that twice the daily requirement of certain amino acids in food leads to toxic cell disturbance, thus $2 \times 35 = 70$ grams. And another study noted; it is as little as 75 grams of daily protein that causes a negative calcium balance (less than three-quarters of what the average meat-eating American consumes).

6. Question #Veg.6   What are reasons people choose to be vegetarians?

About 10-15 million of the U.S. population is vegetarian (depending on how you define it); under 1% of vegetarians in the U.S. are vegan (1997 Roper poll estimated about a million) and probably less than .5% is raw vegan. "An increasing number of people in the United States - between 8.5 and 12.4 million - call themselves vegetarians. At the same time, meatless diets are gaining scientific legitimacy. The American Dietetic Association officially condones vegetarianism. Medical studies support the idea that a healthy diet can be meatless. Yet only about 4% of all vegetarians are vegan.

"People who choose vegetarianism have a variety of reasons for doing so, though research suggests that people's motives vary within rather set categories. In a 1991 survey (Scott 1991), for example, Vegetarian Journal readers revealed their top four reasons: (1) health (reported by 81%), (2) animal rights (81%), (3) ethics (76%), and (4) environment (75%). The other reasons include economics (28%), taste (28%), religion (10%), habit (7%), media articles (8%), friends/family (5%), other (4%), doctor (2%), dietitian (2%). Note that the top four categories reflect the dominant claims in the vegetarian's literature. Four primary motivations emerged from a study of British vegetarians: "moral, health-related, gustatory, and ecological." (1992).

"Other researchers have found similar categories of reasons, and many vegetarians report more than one motive (Amato and Partridge 1989; Beardsworth and Keil 1992; Dwyer et al. 1973; Krizmanic 1992). Four primary motivations emerged from Beardsworth and Keil's study of British vegetarians: "moral, health-related, gustatory, and ecological." The authors note that "in the great majority of instances, respondents had no hesitation in identifying their primary motivation in ways which could be classified quite readily under these headings" (1992).

"The overwhelming majority of vegetarians perceive plant foods as desirable and life-giving (Twigg 1979). By eating food that is more alive, a person becomes healthier. While animal food is considered dead matter, vegetable food lives.

"Most vegetarian authors use scientific evidence to back their arguments. For example, according to John Robbins, "Literally thousands of articles published in the last few decades in The New England Journal of Medicine, the American Journal of Clinical Nutrition, the Journal of the American Medical Association, the British Medical Journal, Lancet, and other publications of similar stature have demonstrated that the less animal fat you take into your body, the healthier you will be" (1992). Richard Bargen, author of the Vegetarian's Self Defense Manual, which reviews over 100 nutritional medical studies, states, "Vegetarianism, once it has achieved a solid scientific foundation, will become the 'norm' in Western nations".

"Scientific data suggest positive relationships between a vegetarian diet and reduced risk for several chronic degenerative diseases and conditions, including obesity, coronary artery disease, hypertension, diabetes mellitus, and some types of cancer." Journal of the American Dietetic Association (Nov. 1997)

"Vegetarians often have lower mortality rates from several chronic degenerative diseases than do nonvegetarians."
British Medical Journal (1996).

7. Question #Veg.7   Do plant-based diets give a longer life?

Yes, plant-based diets give a longer and healthier life then meat-based diets. There is a lot of evidence for this a few comments here will help understand this.

In a medical journal, Dr. Jeremiah Stamler, a cardiologist was talking about lifestyles and demonstrating with statistics on death rate quotes, he noted that: "An additional comparison has recently become available, with data on mortality; for three groups of Californian Seventh Day Adventists (non-vegetarian, lacto-ovo-vegetarian and pure vegetarian) compared with the Californian general population. Seventh Day Adventists have lower mean serum cholesterol levels than Americans generally. For 47,000 Seventh Day Adventist men aged 35 and over, age-sex-standardized, mortality rates were 34% lower for non-vegetarians, 57% lower for the lacto-ovo-vegetarians and 77% lower for the pure vegetarians compared to the general population. Seventh Day Adventists differ from the general population in other respects as well, e.g. abstinence from both alcohol and tobacco."

Dr. Alexander Leaf, chief of medical services at Massachusetts General Hospital in Boston, made an extensive study in three sections of the world where people live extraordinarily long lives: The Andean village of Vilcabamba, Ecuador; the Hunza Kingdom in Kashmir; and the Black Sea coastal area of Abkhazia, in Russia. All of these people were in excellent physical condition. Dr. Leaf's conclusion was that regular physical exercise, heredity, and a sense of importance, in addition to their generally low-calorie and low-protein diets, were important keys to a longer life.

"According to Dr. Alexander Leaf, M.D. who visited the Hunza and made an extensive study of their diet as related to their exceptionally long life, the factors mostly responsible for their long life are: 1) their total low-calorie diet (an average of 1900 calories a day) and 2) their predominantly vegetarian diet (only 1 percent of their protein intake come from animal sources)."

Dr. Leaf says: "I returned from my travels and convinced that vigorous, active old age, free from debility and senility, is possible."

"What can you learn from the Hunza people regarding proteins? Cut down on all proteins, especially animal proteins. The diet with the greatest potential for optimum health and a long life is a lacto-vegetarian diet with emphasis on vegetables, fruits and seeds, nuts and grains, especially in a sprouted form. Homemade cottage cheese (kvark) and soured milk products can supplement this diet, along with vegetable oils and honey. Meat can be left out completely, or the amount consumed reduced drastically."

The average life expectancy in Hunza is between 85 and 90 years and many live to be a healthy 110 to 125. A Dr. Robert McCarrison who lived with the Hunza's for seven years concluded that their traditional diet more than anything else was responsible for their extraordinary health and longevity. Dr. Karl-Otto Aly, a director of a large biological clinic in Sweden did extensive studies on the Hunza people when he visited them. "Their daily diet consists even today of natural, poison-free high quality foods, and is mostly vegetarian. The variety of vegetables and fruits guarantees their adequate supply of various minerals, vitamins, and proteins. The fact that Hunzakuts not only survived in their isolated, rugged mountains, but are enjoying such a high level of health and vitality on such a diet, speaks for its inherent superiority."

Dr. Karl-Otto Aly continued, "According to today's scientific norms and recommendations, the diet of Hunzakuts is utterly protein-deficient, and even deficient in vitamin B12. If we would believe today's orthodox nutritionists, the people of Hunza should have been dead circa 2000 years ago, when they inhabited this isolated river valley and began eating their traditional low animal protein diet. But, apparently not knowing that modern science would not approve of their diet, they fared quite well for over 2000 years. Just like a bumble-bee, which according to all statistical and aerodynamic calculations can't fly, but, being ignorant of the laws of aerodynamics and gravity, flies anyway! Not only did the people of Hunza survive with flying colors, but even today I could not discover a single case of protein deficiency (Kwashiorkor), or anemia and nerve degeneration caused by B12 deficiency."

Dr. Paavo Airola explains that a high protein diet is a sure road to premature aging. "The Hunza example illustrates clearly that it is not a high-protein, but a low-protein diet which has the greatest potential for optimum health and long life. Their average daily intake of protein is about 30 grams. Many other long-living people in the world, like the Russians, Yukatan Indians, Todas, Abhkazians, Vilcabamba inhabitants, and Bulgarians, are people who eat low-protein diets. Hunzakuts eat meat once a month, at the most. According to a recent study of Dr. S. Magsood Ali, of Pakistan, only 1 percent of the Hunzakuts' protein intake was from animal sources. Bulgarians eat very little meat - perhaps 15 - 20 percent of the average American's consumption. In Russia, only 1% percent of the total population are vegetarians, while 9 percent of all people who reach 100 years are vegetarians.

"The healthiest people in Latin America, with the longest life expectancy, are the Yucatan Indians, who never eat meat. Vilcabamba inhabitants in Ecuador show the largest number of centenarians of any place in the world - 1098 for every 100,000 people! According to Dr. Alexander Leaf, M.D., their average protein intake is 35-38 grams a day, and the total caloric intake is only 1200 to 1360 a day. They are almost 100 percent vegetarians."

"The Eskimos and the Lapplanders, who eat very high protein diets of meat, have a life expectancy of 30 -35 years. The Kirgese tribe of Eastern Russia lived primarily on meat and seldom passed the age of 40. Scientists started to correlate diet-styles and health in world populations after World War II. "One fact that emerged consistently was the strong correlation between heavy flesh-eating and short life expectancy. The Eskimos, the Laplanders, the Greenlanders, and the Russian Kurgi tribes stood out as the populations with the highest animal flesh consumption in the world - and also as among the populations with the lowest life expectancies, often only about 30 years. It was found, further, that this was not due to the severity of their climates alone. Other peoples, living in harsh conditions, but subsisting with little or no animal flesh, had some of the highest life expectancies in the world. World health statistics found, for example, that an unusually large number of Russian Caucaians, the Yucatan Indians, the East Indian Todas and the Pakistan Hunzakuts have life expectancies of 90 to 100 years." (*Diet for a New America*)

"The cultures with the very longest life spans in the world are the Vilcambas, who reside in the Andes of Ecuador, the Abkhasians, who live on the Black Sea in the USSR, and the Hunzas, who live in the Himalayas of Northern Pakistan. Researchers discovered a 'striking similarity' in the diets of these groups, scattered though they are in different parts of the plant. All three are either totally vegetarian or close to it." (Diet for a New America)

8. Question #Veg.8 What is the longest known life-span of a person in modern times?

Dr. Paavo Airola reports that the renowned Chinese scholar and herbalist, Professor Li Chung Yun, who lived to be 265 years of age. Don't laugh! Professor Li Chung Yun's age is well documented. Being a world-famous scholar, he was in the public eye for over 200 years. At the age of 100, he was awarded by the Chinese government a special Honor Citation for extraordinary services to his country. This document is available in existing archives. For over 150 years after the award, the Professor was visited by countless Western scholars and students. It is reported that he gave a series of 28 lectures at the University of Sinkiang when he was over 200 years old.

His life spanned four centuries - 16th, 17th, 18th, and 19th. He enjoyed excellent health, outlived 23 wives, and kept his own natural teeth and hair. Those who saw him at the age of 200 testified that he did not appear much older than a man in his fifties. Professor Li Chung Yun attributed his longevity to his life-long vegetarian diet and the regular use of rejuvenating herbs plus - may I add, an important plus - to his "inward calm". He used gotu-kola (hydrocotyle asiatica minor) and ginseng daily in the form of tea.

Researchers and writers who studied his life in detail, attributed his long life to his vegetarian diet and special rejuvenate herb teas which he drank all of his life: ginseng and got-kola. Li Chung Yun himself, however, had a different idea for the reason of his long life. When asked to what he attributed his long life, he said: "I attribute my long life to INWARD CALM."

Dr. Paavo Airola states, "In all my studies of people who lived extraordinarily long lives in various parts of the world, I have found that in addition to all the other factors, such as sound nutrition of simple, unadulterated foods, scanty eating, poison free environment, and plenty of exercise, they all possessed that unmistakable quality Professor Yun was taking about - INWARD CALM." A more conservative estimate of Li Ching-Yun's age placed him at 197 years old, born in 1783.

9. Question # Veg.9 What are some scientific reasons for this long lifespan?

Dr. Paavo Airola also gives a scientific reason why a low intake of protein is connected to a long life. "A high animal protein diet, is one of the main causes of senility and premature aging which has been recently stressed by two leading European biochemists and doctors - Professor Ph. Schwarz, of Frankfurt University, and Dr. Ralph Bircher of Zurich, Switzerland. They reported that the aging processes are triggered by a substance called amyloid, a by-product of protein metabolism, which is deposited in connective tissues and causes tissue and organ degeneration. Amyloid, the aging-producing substance, contains a large percentage of the amino acids tryptophan and tyrosine, which are plentiful in animal proteins. 'The connection between deposits of amyloid in the tissues and the degenerative diseases and aging processes in man has been known for a long time, but conveniently forgotten in this age of the high protein fad.' Famous German pathologist, Dr. Rudolf Virchow, suggested as early as 1854 that amyloid deposits cause degenerative changes and premature aging. Amyloidosis was produced in experimental animals by feeding them high-protein diets."

It is interesting if we go back to the Biblical Account of the Flood where God first allowed man to eat meat and also said his life span would be only 120 years, whereas before it was over 800 years old. On a strict vegetarian diet with fruit and vegetable based protein this amyloid problem is minimized, but with meat it is accentuated. Perhaps God was aware of this?

It should be stated that a vegetarian diet is an alkaline diet and all the longest lived populations had this alkaline diet. Most all the major nature oriented healing centers use an alkaline based diet to heal major illness. Man's pH is 7.43 which is slightly on the alkaline side and sickness usually happens when the body chemistry is in an acid state. The

Standard American Diet (meat eaters) are on the acid side of the pH scale.

10. Question #Veg.10 What are other scientific evidence for long life spans?

A Dr. Edward Stiegbitz in his book, The Second Forty Years, points out that: "Superficially, the answer is simple; intrinsically, extremely complex.... The quality of the cellular environment is the determining factor, whether the cells be growing in vitro in a test-tube, in vivo, or in the living and functioning organism."

The plant-based writer Ross Horne comments on these and other hypothesis on old age: "So it becomes clear that "old-age" occurs because we take into our bodies, mainly in food, harmful substances which overtax the digestive system, cause toxemia of the milieu interieur, overtax the eliminatory organs, and to a greater or lesser extent in the form of foreign compounds, gradually accumulate in the tissues and cells to increasingly impede their functions. It follows then that old-age can be deferred by selecting foods which provide the best nutrition with the least digestive effort and the least amount of harmful residues, and consuming such foods in great moderation."

One scientific study showed that fasting (diet restriction) is the only consistently proven method of extending lifespan and this article hypothesizes that it is because it reduces the total amount of oxidative stress within an animal. Technically speaking: Oxygen destroys mitochondrial genomes which lack DNA repair mechanisms. Diet restriction can attenuate age associate mitochondrial enzymatic dysfunction. People who fast and eat a Live-Food diet will probably live longer, this goes along with the moderation as a factor that is found in people who live over a hundred years.

The research done cross culturally with groups like the

Hunza people and within the U.S. with groups like the 7th Day Adventists, tends to indicate that a strict vegetarian diet is the healthiest and gives the longest life span. The doctors and practitioners of a raw vegan or Live-Food diet has the highest healing rates of degenerative diseases.

Meat Based Diets
(Ani. means animals)

11. Question #Ani.11   Are their differences between humans and animals?

Yes, there are very clear physiological differences between humans and animals in relation to the foods that we eat. The diet of an animal usually relates to its physiological structure. There are meat eating animals and non-meat eating or vegetarian (grass and leaf) eating animals. And there are a few animals like the apes that are fruit and nut eating animals. Apes are the strongest animals on earth for their size. A silver-back gorilla has 30 times the strength and only 3 times the size of man. These gorillas eat nothing but fruit and bamboo leaves and can turn your car over if they wanted to.

a) Meat Eating Animals
1) has claw, to rip flesh;
2) no pores on the skin, perspires through tongue to cool body;
3) it has sharp front canine teeth, no flat molar teeth;
4) no flat back molar teeth;
5) small salivary glands in the front of the mouth;
6) acid saliva with no enzyme ptyalin;
7) strong hydrochloric acid in the stomach to digest meat;
8) intestinal track is smooth and only 3 times the body length which helps pass decaying meat quickly.
9) urine is acidic from meat eating diet;
10) liver contains enzymes to break down uric acid.

b) Vegetarian Animals, Apes and Humans
1) no claws but hands with nails to pick and peel fruits;
2) perspires through pores on skin;
3) no sharp front canine teeth for tearing meat;
4) flat, back molar teeth to grind food;
5) well-developed salivary glands which are used to pre-digest grains and fruits;
6) alkaline saliva with enzyme ptyalin to pre-digest grains;
7) stomach acid about 20 times weaker then the meat eating animals;
8) intestinal track is puckered and 10 times the body length for veggie animals and 12 times body length for apes and humans.
9) urine is alkaline from vegetarians and fruits (average person)
10) liver has a low tolerance for uric acid.

The gorilla is the strongest land mammal in the world (pound for pound). The gorilla could lift about 3 to 4,000 pounds if it needed to. The gorilla is a strict vegetarian, more than that the gorilla is a raw vegetarian, who eats a lot of leafy green vegetables and fruit.

The original, natural and best foods for humans is probably fruits. Of all the animals on the earth we are more closely related to the friutivous animals, the fruitarian animals. Humans are not closely related to the herbivores, the cows, the horses, etc. Man is not a natural grass eater by nature. Our jaws do not chew with a four way action: back and forth and up and down, like tritration with the jaws to grin the grasses down and extract the juices, as herbivores do. And we do not have double and triple stomachs to flip the foods back and forth and get the most out of greens.

Animal intestines can handle the putrefying bacteria, high levels of fat and lack of fiber and intestinal acid since their intestine is designed for it. "The digestion of meat itself produces strong carcinogenic substances in the colon and meat-eaters must produce extensive bile acids in their intestines to deal with the meat they eat, particularly deoxycholic acid. This is extremely significant, because deoxycholic acid is converted by clostridia bacteria in our intestines into powerful carcinogens. The fact that meat-eaters invariably have far more deoxycholic acid in their intestines than do vegetarians is one of the reasons they have so much higher rates of colon cancer." (American Journal of Digestive Diseases, (1975), Journal of Pathology, (1971))

A paper presented to the "American Heart Association" council on atherosclerosis states: "Examination of the dental structure of modern man reveals that he possesses all of the features of a strictly herbivorous animal. While designed to subsist on vegetarian foods, he has perverted his dietary to accept the food of the carnivore. It is postulated that man cannot handle carnivorous food like the carnivore. Herein may lie the basis for the high incidence of human atherosclerotic disease."

The medical journal Lancet reports: "Formerly, vegetable proteins were classified as second-class, and regarded as inferior to first-class proteins of animal origin, but this distinction has now been generally discarded." The Food and Nutrition Board of the National Academy of Sciences notes: "Pure vegetarians from many populations of the world have maintained... excellent health."

12. Question #Ani.12   Are high protein meat-based diets dangerous?

Studies are consistently showing that high protein consumption also means higher rates of cancer development. "T. Colin Campbell, a Professor of Nutritional Sciences at Cornell University and the senior science advisor to the American Institute for Cancer Research, says there is 'a strong correlation between dietary protein intake and cancer of the breast, prostate, pancreas and colon.'" Professor Campbell goes on in his book, The China Study, to show study after study that shows plant-based diets are superior to meat-based diets.

Likewise, Myron Winick, director of Columbia University's Institute of Human Nutrition, has found strong evidence of "a relationship between high-protein diets and cancer of the colon.'

In Your Health, Your Choice, Dr. Morter writes, "The paradox of protein is that it is not only essential but also potentially health-destroying. Adequate amounts are vital keeping your cells hale and hearty and on the job; but unrelenting consumption of excess dietary protein congests your cells and forces the pH of your life-sustaining fluids down to cell-stifling, disease-producing levels. Cells overburdened with protein become toxic."

Two journal studies showed that excess protein can cause a fluid imbalance and result in kidney damage. "The liver and kidneys are the organs called upon to change excess protein, and too much work puts a strain on them. Because of this extra work the body heat level is raised and the fluid balance is upset. A continued excess may result in damage to the kidneys."
("Observations on Nitrogen and Energy Balance in Young Men Consuming Vegetarian Diets," American Journal of Clinical Nutrition; "High Protein Ration as a Cause of Nephritis," California and Western Medicine).

See Question # Ani.28 for a list of some dangers of excess protein. In summary: excess fat and excess cholesterol promotes tumor growth; rise in serum cholesterol; possible toxic nitrogen by-products; Ammonia is carcinogenic and urea promotes arthritis; meat-based diets, are acidic; incidence of osteoporosis correlates directly with protein intake; adverse effects of excessive protein intake on calcium loss; Amyloid deposits cause degenerative changes thus a shorter lifespan and premature aging from excess protein; Cooking meat creates mutagens which alters the DNA; excess protein can be damaging to the kidneys; diets high in animal protein increase one's risk of kidney stones and gallstones.

13. Question # Ani.13   Does high protein clog the membranes?

The Wendt doctrine, explains one major factor connecting excess protein consumption to some forms of chronic degenerative disease like MS and PD. The Wendts were able to prove with electron microscope pictures that excess protein clogs the basement membrane, a filtering membrane located between capillaries and cells. It helps regulate the flow of nutrients and waste products between capillaries, cells, and fluid in the tissues they penetrate. The more excess protein there is lodged in the basement membrane, results in a thicker basement membrane with clogged pores. It becomes harder for proteins, other nutrients, and even oxygen to get through into the cells and for waste and breakdown products to get out of the cells. This could be a major part of the problem and milk and dairy products would be involved in this build-up leading to many degenerative diseases.

The Wendt doctrine, is a result of thirty years of research by Wendt, Wendt, and Wendt, a family of physician researchers, has now received formal recognition by nutritional scientists in Germany. It explains one major factor connecting excess protein consumption to some forms of chronic degenerative disease.

"The Wendts were able to prove with electron microscope pictures that excess protein clogs the basement membrane, a filtering membrane located between capillaries and cells. It helps regulate the flow of nutrients and waste products between capillaries, cells, and fluid in the tissues they penetrate. Excess protein lodges in the basement membrane, resulting in a thicker basement membrane/clogged pores. It becomes harder for proteins, other nutrients, and even oxygen to get through into the cells and also harder for waste and breakdown products to get out of the cells. Eventually, the basement membrane becomes so clogged with excess protein that the cells on the inside of the capillary walls begin to store and secrete the excess protein in insoluble forms that accumulate on the inside of the capillaries and arteriole walls, causing atherosclerosis, hypertension, adult-onset diabetes, and what the Wendts term capillarogenic tissue degeneration, the result of clogged basement membranes all over the system."

"This clogged basement membrane produces cellular malnutrition and results in the anoxia of the tissues. According to Dr. Steven Levine's hypothesis, anoxia is the cause of all degenerative diseases. The key understanding is that excess protein in the diet results in a protein storage disease that slowly chokes off the system. It is much harder to meditate when one is choking on a cellular level and the vitality of the system is slowly dying out. The Wendts found that this whole process could be reversed by stopping the intake of all animal protein for one to three months, and by eating a low-protein diet or by doing extensive fasting."

14. Question # Ani.14 Does the stress in animals influence the meat?

Not only the food the animal eats affects us but studies have shown that stress on the animal causes biochemical changes: "This metabolic responsiveness to stress alters its composition and thus cannot fail to affect its nature as meat." Thus we become part of what we eat including the stress." (The Physiology and Biochemistry of Muscle as Food, Univ. of Wisconsin Press)

Animals go through a great deal of stress during the last few days of their life and right before they are killed, slaughter houses are awful places of killing hundreds of animals a day. This stress goes into the meat, then the animals are killed and it stays in the meat.

15. Question # Ani.15   What about the question of antibiotics?

About half of the 31 million pounds of antibiotics produced every year in the U.S. goes into animal feed to make them fatter. "Because of health concerns over antibiotic-resistant bacteria, several European countries banned the use of antibiotics in animal feed in the 1970's. Our government is still dragging its feet due to money, power and politics."

Animals are given antibiotic-laced feeds to help make them fatter and not just because they may be sick. About half of the 31 million pounds of antibiotics produced every year in the U.S. goes into animal feed. About 80% of the poultry and 75% of the pigs get antibiotics to make them bigger. "Because of health concerns over antibiotic-resistant bacteria, several European countries banned the use of antibiotics in animal feed in the 1970's. Our government is still dragging its feet due to money, power and politics, not science! Besides penicillin and tetracycline in meat, you also can get nitrofurazone (and other nitrofurans), and sulfamethazine (along with other sulfa drugs). These can increase the risk of cancer."

Until about the 1960's, meat was a largely uncontaminated product. Few chemicals found their way into the chops, steaks and roasts you put on your table. But today, one of the fastest-growing - and most potentially dangerous - developments in agriculture is the use of a host of new chemicals in feed, livestock medication and meat processing. A past headline points up the new trend: 'Livestock Thrive on Chemical Diet.' Like a whirlwind, chemical feeding is taking over. The animals and poultry we eat have become as chemicalized as the plant products now on the market.

The meat of poultry is the same muscle fiber as the meat of beef and has the same acidity. Stay away from beef but if for some reason you have to eat poultry, eat organic poultry, free range, which does not have these hormones and chemicals.

Wolfe; Arlin; Dini, in Nature's First Law, point out: Chlorinated hydrocarbon pesticide residues in the U.S. diet: Supplied by meat. 55%; Supplied by dairy products: 23% ; Suppied by vegetables: 6% ; Supplied by fruits: 4% ; Supplied by grains: 1% ; Percentage of U.S. mother's milk containing significant levels of DDT: 99% ; Percentage of U.S. vegetarian mother's milk containing significant levels of DDT: 8% ; Relative pesticide contamination in breast milk of meat-eating mothers compared to pesticide contamination in breast milk of vegetarian mothers: 35 times as high; Percentage of male college students sterile in 1950: 0.5%; Percentage of male college students sterile in 1978: 25%; Sperm count of an average American male compared to 35 years ago: Down 30%; Principle reason for sterility and sperm count reduction of U.S. males; Chlorinated hydrocarbon pesticides (including dioxin, DDT, etc.); Percentage of hydrocarbon pesticide residues in American diet attributable to meats, dairy products, fish, and eggs: 94%. Less than 1 out of every 250,000 slaughtered animals is tested for toxic chemical residues."

16. Question # Ani.16 What about eating poultry?

Of the major types of disease-causing bacteria and parasites found in food, nearly all have been found in meat or poultry. "Poultry in America is commonly contaminated with salmonella. The USDA says that about one-third of raw chickens are contaminated with salmonella. But some unbiased experts say 50 to 90 percent of poultry leaving the plant are contaminated. In 1990, the University of Wisconsin screened over 2,300 laying hens from three flocks. They found only eight birds that were not infected with campylobacter, another "bug" that causes food poisoning."

"Poultry seems particularly prone to contamination with

campylobacters; 80% of chickens and 90% of turkeys carried through a typical slaughterhouse produced positive cultures for it. Complete cooking can kill most of these microbes and bacteria that are found in poultry. But campylobacters survive freezing and "chicken that appears pink and underdone is the most likely source of infection." Thus sandwiches and salads that have chicken and turkey meat without being cooked properly should be avoided.

Inspectors inspect chickens at a rate of one every two seconds or so, as they speed by the inspectors on hooks. But these inspections do not detect bacterial, antibiotic or other chemicals or toxin contamination. The USDA only uses tests that detect about 40 of the 227 different pesticides used on meat.

"Before 1950, antibiotics were not used but today chickens have a steady supply of sulfa drugs, hormones, antibiotics and nitrofurans. Veterinary drugs are used on every food-producing animal and many of these thousands of new drugs have not been tested. Over 90% of the chickens today are fed arsenic compounds." One of the dyes injected into chickens is used so that their meat and yolks will appear to be a "healthy looking" yellow.

Gabriel Cousens, MD, notes: According to the Project Censored ratings, a news report in the June 8, 1990 Pacific Sun, the "fowl" play in the chicken industry was voted one of the ten most underreported stories of 1989. In their article it is pointed out that the incidence of bacterial salmonella infection is now two and one-half million cases per year, including an estimated one-half million hospitalizations and nine thousand deaths. Apparently the epidemic is caused by a huge leap in consumer demand for "healthier food" called chicken, as they switch from red meat, and by a massive failure of the US Department of Agriculture to inspect the chicken. A decrease in USDA staff led to an increase in contaminated chicken slipping through en masse. The article states: The USDA has placed gag orders on inspectors and destroyed documents disclosing that the agency has approved massive amounts of contaminated food. In the Pacific Sun article, Dr. Carl Telleen, a retired USDA veterinarian revealed how …chicken carcasses contaminated with feces, once routinely condemned or trimmed, are now simply rinsed with chlorinated water to remove stains. According to Telleen, Thousands of dirty chickens are bathed together in a chill tank, creating a mixture known as "fecal soup" that spreads contamination from bird to bird. This creates what Telleen calls "instant sewage." (*Conscious Eating*).

17. Question # Ani.17 What about eating turkey instead of chickens?

"You may wonder whether you'd be better off eating turkey. Sorry, but the methods applied to the factory production of poultry and eggs are also applied to other birds, such as turkeys, geese and ducks. All these birds are treated with equal disdain for their natural urges and needs, and equal fixation on using them for profit. They are debeaked, stuffed in wire cages, and fed the same sort of unnatural diet as chickens, complete with chemicals, drugs, and antibiotics."

Neil Bernard, MD notes: "Breaking a meat habit cuts your overall cancer risk by about 40 percent. Your risk of colon cancer drops by about two-thirds, according to Harvard University studies including tens of thousands of women and men." (*British Medical Journal; New England Journal Medicine*)

18. Question #Veg.18   What about eating fish?

A century ago fish was a healthy source of food but today eating fish is questionable and problematic because of the mercury, chemicals and heavy metals from pollution. However, fish is a much healthier food to eat then beef and poultry. But there is a good side and bad side to eating fish.

Because of the greenhouse effect and the warming of the climate, there has been an increase in parasites and bacterial in the fresh waters thus it is better not to eat fish raw. Cooking fish will kill most parasites and bacteria, and those that it does not kill are not going to harm you.

Some sources have indicated that as much as 70 milligrams of mercury can kill a person. Some deep-sea fish, such as blue-fin tuna and swordfish, and even some California game fish, contain half a milligram of mercury for every kilo (2.2 pounds) of their body weight. It is easy to see that if a person were to eat such fish at the rate most Americans eat beef, the lethal limit would be reached in only five or six years."

Neal Barnard, MD, founder of The Physician's Committee for Responsible Medicine in Washington, D.C. who writes that: "Many people have turned from red meats to fish, encouraged by reports that fish contains "good fats." However, those "good fats" are just as fattening as any other kind of fat, as the native populations of Arctic regions have demonstrated. Perhaps the worst of all, fish is by far the most contaminated food. As environmental experts monitor chemical contamination in fish, they routinely issue advisories, such as one from Virginia's Department of Environment Quality, which recently pointed out that catfish and carp had PCBs up to 3,212 parts per billion, more than five times the allowable limit. PCBs, or polychlorinated biphenyls, are chemicals that were used in electrical equipment, hydraulic fluid, and carbonless carbon paper. They linger in waterways and, like mercury and other contaminants, flow through fish gills, lodge in fish muscle tissues, and routinely show up in governmental tests."

Brian Clement, PhD writes in his book, Killer Fish that, "There are three central reasons why one should not be eating fish and other aquatic life. First' is the fact that these creatures harbor saturated fats and disease-causing elements derived from the way we prepare them for consumption. Next, is the fact that each of these creatures is filled with our industrial waste (chemicals, heavy metals, etc.) and the globally scattered radiation from our endless wars and faulty nuclear energy endeavors? Last, but not least, are the multitude of parasites and amoebas that water-based creatures contain, which are passed to those unfortunate individuals who eat them."

19. Question # Ani.19   What about getting omega 3 and 6 from fish?

Brian Clement, PhD writes in his book, Killer Fish that; "Fish gives the wrong ratio of these fats and creates an imbalance of omega 3 to 6. Dr. Clement points out that, 'There is often an 11:1 ratio of omega-6/omega-3 in some of the most commonly consumed fish versus the optimum 1:3 level found in plant-based sources. The unhealthy fatty acid ratio found in many common fish precipitates higher levels of cardiovascular disease for those who consistently eat these 'fishy foods.'

"Another common myth is that fish oil slows mental decline. A study from the Journal of the American Medical Association (JAMA) reports that there was no benefit derived by a group consuming fish oil since their cognitive function did not improve mild to moderate Alzheimer's disease. JAMA went on to say, 'There is no basis for recommendation of supplementation in the quest of helping those afflicted with dementia.'"

Finally, Dr. Clement writes about the long legacy of people who have contracted disease by consuming aquatic life. He writes "The handful of studies that point to fish as a heart-healthy food are over-shadowed by many studies that prove their consumption actually severely increase the chances of heart attacks and strokes. As far back as 2004, Annals of Internal Medicine stated, 'Americans have heard less about, and have paid less attention to, various health warnings associated with fish consumption. Studies have linked overconsumption of certain popular fish to neurological deficits, cancer, auto-immune and endocrine disorders, and in addition, heart disease.'"

20. Question Ani.20 What about eating fish rather than red meat?

I do need to be honest that there are two opinions of eating fish, Brian Clement, PhD has expressed one in the last two questions in his book, Killer Fish. Another opinion emphasizes that some studies show eating fish has been shown to be healthier then eating red meat. An important study was written up in a Scandinavian medical journal which compared Greenlanders to their counterparts in Denmark, both of which have the same Nordic background and similar genetic makeup. The diets were very similar but Greenlanders lived on the coast and ate mostly fish while the Danes ate mostly meat. The Greenlanders were much healthier then the Danes. The Greenlanders had no incidence of Diabetes, Asthma, Multiple Sclerosis, Inflammatory Bowel Disease or Breast Cancer, while the Danes had high or very high incidences of these diseases. The Greenlanders had a measurable, but very small level, of Heart Attack, Psoriasis, Thyroid Toxicosis and Rheumatoid arthritis whereas the Danes had very high incidences of these diseases. Other diseases; like Ulcers, Cancer and Epilepsy were much less in the Greenlanders. Comparisons can be made with:
- Canadians in maritime provinces, where cold-water fish is a dietary staple, have much less rheumatoid arthritis and inflammatory disease in general.
- Italians who live inland with a diet rich in meat, have more rheumatoid arthritis, versus whose who live on the seacoast and eat fish and vegetables.
- Asians who migrate to the United States and take on our meat-oriented diet, have more rheumatoid arthritis, compared to siblings who remain in Asia and eat a more vegetarian and fish-oriented die,
- Japanese who live in seacoast villages and eat a diet rich in

fish and almost completely exclude meat have much less rheumatoid arthritis compared to inland villagers who eat meat.

- The most recent research indicates these same patterns hold for multiple sclerosis, which is also an inflammatory autoimmune disease with many similarities to rheumatoid arthritis.

The magnitude of the differences were not always the same, but the trends were consistent: eating fish rather than meat matters.

21. Question # Ani.21 What about eating fresh water fish?

Dr. Eric R. Brown, chairman of the microbiology department of the Chicago Medical School went fishing with his son one day. Curious about the tumors on the fish he caught, Dr. Brown initiated an investigation of the fish and of the water where he was fishing - Fox River, a typical American river flowing a few miles west of Chicago. The bacteria count ran as high as 39,000 per 100 milliliters of water. That indicated a high proportion of fecal matter. There were also herbicides, insecticides, phosphates, nitrates, gasoline, ether, and carcinogenic (cancer-producing compounds of the benzathracene group) substances. In addition, lead, mercury, calcium, cadmium, zinc, and antimony were found.

"What a fish eats of elements such as mercury and arsenic, Dr. Brown points out, the fish keeps. When a bigger fish eats several smaller fish, he keeps the mercury and arsenic that they all ate. When a human being eats the fish, he keeps these poisons and they build up in him. This process of 'biological magnification' is a major threat in the use of flesh as food." The lethal limit for mercury poisoning would be reached in only five or six years by a person eating some types of fish at the rate most Americans eat beef.

Do you want to play Russian roulette and take chances eating fish? There is mercury in almost all fish and some levels are called 'acceptable' according to the government. Why gamble? Just avoid fish!

In the book: The Brain Gate, Robert Hatherill, PhD, notes: "Fish and shellfish contain mercury (methylmercury), and mercury vapors have been demonstrated to cross the BrainGate. Once mercury crosses the BrainGate, a number of toxic processes occur. Mercury creates oxidative stress by depleting antioxidants. This depletion then blocks the formation of the brain messenger acetylcholine. The decrease in acetylcholine occurs mostly in the brain cortex and hippocampus." In addition, Dr. Hatherill continues: "High levels of homocysteine result primarily from the intake of animal proteins, not plant proteins. Animal proteins contain an abundance of the essential amino acid methionine. If you eat a lot of methionine-rich foods, you will form higher levels of the toxic amino acid homocysteine. Homocysteine is formed from methionine. Fish have particularly high levels of methionine. To convert toxic homocysteine back into methionine requires folic acid and B vitamins. Some researchers believe that it's elevated homocysteine levels, and not high cholesterol, that actually cause brain strokes."

22. Question # Ani.22   What about Mad Cow disease in meat?

"About 75 percent of the ninety million beef cattle in America are routinely given feed that has been 'enriched' with rendered animal parts. The use of animal excrement in feed is common as well, as livestock operators have found it to be an efficient way of disposing of a portion of the 1.6 million tons of livestock wastes generated annually by their industry. If you are a meat-eater, understand that this is the food of your food."

Mad Cow disease or 'BSE' or CJD the human equivalent (which turns the brain to mush) is because of animals eating other animals put in their feed. The disease has been found in

20 different animals and 12 or more countries. The disease is impervious to high temperatures (680 degrees F), drying and freezing, most disinfectants, and radiation. The incubation period takes two to eight years in a cow before the cow shows any signs of having it. CJD is very similar to Alzheimer's and one report found 50 out of 66 Alzheimer's patients with CJD. Like HIV it can be transmitted through milk. These diseases are fatal, and found in meats.

(A few of the key references for the above facts include: *J Infect Dis* 1990; Freezing - World Health Organization Fact sheet: Bovine Spongiform Encephalopathy (BSE); U.S. Department of Agriculture, 1996; Creutzfeldt-Jakob disease with Alzheimer... *Histopathology* 1995; Vacuolar change in Alzheimer's disease, *Arch Neurol* 1987; Creutzfeldt-Jokob disease, *N Eng J Med* 1992.)

23. Question # Ani.23   What about animal protein pathogenic microorganisms?

It should be noted that the average American meal of animal products contains 750,000,000 - 1,000,000,000 pleomorphic pathogenic microorganisms per meal (US Department of Agriculture). The average vegetarian meal, consisting of only plant food has less than 500 pleomorphic pathogenic microorganisms per meal. The body's defense system can easily handle this low amount, but the higher amounts indicated above for animal products are problematic especially for neurological diseases like Parkinson's, MS, Alzheimer's or ALS. A plant-based diet is obviously healthier because it contains less pathogenic microorganisms per meal. These are unhealthy microorganisms, something the body does not need or want. The brain also does not need or want this influence which could lead to numerous problems such as fungi in the brain and Lewy bodies found in Parkinson's and MS. Let us look at this chart."

"This chart shows Animal Foods for acceptable sale per U.S. Department of Agriculture
• Milk, Grade A Pasteurized: 20,000 microorganisms/

pathogens per gram, or 5,000,000 per cup.
• Butter: 300,000 to 1,000,000 microorganisms/ pathogens per gram, or 7,000,000 per patty.
• Cheese: 300,000 to 1,000,000 microorganisms/ pathogens per gram, or 100,000,000 per serving.
• Ice Cream: 300,000 to 1,000,000 microorganisms/ pathogens per gram, or 225,000,000 per serving.
• Eggs: 50,000 to 500,000 microorganisms/pathogens per gram, or 37,500,000 per egg.
• Beef, Poultry, Lamb, Pork, Seafood: 300,000 to 3,000,000 microorganisms/pathogens per gram, or 336,000,000 per serving.
• Honey: 500,000 microorganisms/pathogens per gram.

¬ The average American meal of animal products contains 750,000,000 - 1,000,000,000 pleomorphic pathogenic microorganisms per meal (US Department of Agriculture).
¬ The average vegetarian meal consisting of only plant food has less than 500 pleomorphic pathogenic microorganisms per meal. The body's defense system can easily handle this low amount, but the higher amounts indicated above for animal products are problematic, and for some with diseases dangerous.
Vegetables, fruits, legumes, seeds, nuts and sprouted grains (if uncontaminated in handling): are only 10 microorganisms/ pathogens per gram.

24. Question # Ani.24 What about milk and dairy products?

Cows milk is for Cows. It helps them grow to 1,500 lbs.! Goats milk is actually the same pH and close to the same nutrients as mothers milk. If you have to choose milk choose goats milk and goats milk products over cow's milk.

Dr. Frank A. Oski, M.D. Director, Department of Pediatrics, John Hopkins School of Medicine states: "It is estimated that half the iron-deficiency in infants in the United States is primarily a result of cow's milk inducing gastrointestinal bleeding. This is a staggering figure when one realizes that approximately 15 to 20 percent of all children under the age of two in this country suffer from iron-deficiency anemia. The resultant iron-deficiency anemia makes the child irritable, apathetic, and inattentive. The infant cries a great deal, the mother gives a bottle of milk to soothe him, and the condition continues to get worse. (*Pediatrics*)

"Diarrhea and cramps, gastrointestinal bleeding, iron-deficiency anemia, skin rashes, atherosclerosis, and acne. These are disorders that have been linked to the drinking of whole cow milk. So have recurrent ear infections and bronchitis. Yes. Leukemia, multiple sclerosis, rheumatoid arthritis, and simple dental decay have also been proposed. In one study on multiple sclerosis in the United States, they also studied twenty one other nations and the only significant link was between multiple sclerosis and average milk consumption." (*Lancet*)

Another study found an apparent relationship between heavy milk drinking and anti-social behavior. "It was found that the juvenile delinquents consumed almost ten times the amount of milk that was drunk by the control group. Possibly the consumption of large quantities of milk produced some form of 'protein intoxication' that resulted in crime. 'Who knows what evil lurks in the minds (or stomachs) of men?' " (J Ortho Psych) Dr. H.L. Newbold, a psychiatrist, has identified many patients in his practice whose insomnia, anxiety, or depression has been produced by foods. The food most responsible for the symptoms in both adults and children is whole cow milk." (*Pediatr Clin No Amer*)

Dr. Robert Young PhD. points out, "The idea that dairy products are healthy is pure hype and a cultural myth. While cheese is a product of fermentation, dairy foods also contain residues of hormones and fungally based antibiotics, as well as yeast, fungus, mold, and mycotoxins (cows are fed stored grains). Dairy is also the leader of all foods in being mucoid-forming. It just gums you up. In addition, milk and especially cheese contain lactose (milk sugar). Eight ounces of milk have approximately twelve grams of lactose that can break down into yeast, fungus - feeding sugars. If all that isn't enough, pasteurization destroys any enzymes that might be there to begin with, and makes the milk "sick". Sick milk will rot and stink if left out, proving that pasteurization doesn't even work (can't kill microzymas), whereas raw milk will curdle naturally, and is still 'edible.' Last but not least, dairy is highly acid-forming. Add the influence of a variety of refined sugars to the above, and you've got a real winner: ice cream." (Young, Robert, O., Sick and Tired)

In Robert Cohen's book, Milk A-Z. The book shows how milk can be the cause of: allergies; breast cancer; Crohn's disease; diabetes; ear infections; fat; growth hormones; heart disease; iron deficiency; juvenile illnesses; killer bacteria; lactose intolerance; mad cow disease; nasal congestion; osteoporosis; pesticide intake; rheumatoid arthritis; sudden infant death; tuberculosis; uterine cancer; vitamin D problems; and zits.

Robert Hatherhill PhD in his book BrainGate, explains that studies show that milk consumption increases lead and cadmium absorption. The main protein in milk, casein, has been shown to increase lead levels in the brains, liver, and kidneys of animals. Researchers have not determined why this happens, but it is possible that heavy metals piggyback on the amino acids in milk to get access to the brain. Milk fat also increases uptake of lead and other environmental pollutants.'"

While daily calcium intake is important, numerous studies have clearly demonstrated that too much dietary protein, not too little calcium, is the major cause of osteoporosis. Why? Too much protein causes an excess of hydrogen ions in the blood, which elevates blood acid levels. Because high acid levels can be dangerous, the body 'buffers,' or neutralizes the blood acid levels by drawing calcium from the bones. The resulting waste products, including calcium, are excreted in the urine. This evidence can be found in various journals including: *American Journal of Clinical Nutrition, Journal of Nutrition, Journal of the American Dietetic Association, and Hospital Practice.*

"Another author states: 'Even the most conservative medical investigators no longer deny the connection between excess protein and osteoporosis. In a report published in the British journal Lancet, Drs. Aaron Watchman and Daniel Bernstein commented on work sponsored by the United States Department of Health and Harvard University. They called the association of meat-based diets with the increasing incidence of osteoporosis 'inescapable.'" (Lancet)

In his book, *The BrainGate*, Dr. Hatherill, PhD an expert on brain toxins explains:
• Milk increases the uptake of neurotoxic cadmium, mercury, and lead in the brain.
• The milk sugar galactose builds up in the lens of the eye, causing cataracts.
• Dairy products create an increased risk of diabetes. Diabetics are developing more serious nervous system problems, such as dementia.
• The high fat content of dairy products leads to increased intake of neurotoxic environmental chemicals like PCB and dioxin.
• Milk causes leaky gut, which does not support optimal brain health.
• Milk intake increases heart disease risk, which ultimately impacts brain function."

Every single study in history that has been done on Parkinson's and dairy found that the more dairy products consumed, the higher the risk of getting Parkinson's. So a meta-analysis of all prospective studies on dairy/milk consumption and the risk of Parkinson's disease in men and woman were done and they found that dairy consumption was positively associated with the risk of Parkinson's disease. (*Am J Epidemiol*)

"Studies have suggested that bovine serum albumin is the milk protein responsible for the onset of diabetes." (New England Journal of Medicine) "These new studies, and more than 20 well-documented previous ones, have prompted one researcher to say the link between milk and juvenile diabetes is 'very solid'." (*Diabetes Care*)

Lactose is a milk sugar and most adults lack the enzyme, lactase which breaks down lactose. "An estimated 50 million Americans experience intestinal discomfort after consuming dairy products. Symptoms include bloating, stomach pain, cramps, gas, or diarrhea." (*American Journal of Epidemiology; Postgraduate Medicine*)

In the countries where dairy products are consumed the greatest (United States, Finland, Sweden and the United Kingdom) osteoporosis is found to be most common. (*American Journal of Clinical Nutrition; also Nutrition Action Healthletter*)

"Preference for a diet high in animal fat could be a pathogenic factor, and milk and high fat dairy products contribute considerably to dietary fat intake." Journal of the American College of Nutrition "Milk and milk products gave the highest correlation coefficient to heart disease, while sugar, animal proteins and animal fats came in second, third and fourth, respectively." Medical Hypothesis - Survey of mortality rates in 24 countries.

According to the microbiologist Dr. Robert Young, PhD, D.Sc., "an increase in lactose (a sugar) from dairy products, especially cheese and ice cream, increases the lactic acid in the body which ferments in the bowels, the blood and the brain, leading to Parkinson's and other neurological diseases. He points out, the idea that dairy products are healthy is pure hype and a cultural myth. While cheese is a product of fermentation, dairy foods also contain residues of hormones and fungally-based antibiotics, as well as yeast, fungus, mold, and mycotoxins because cows are fed stored grains. Dairy is also the leader of all foods in being mucoid-forming. It just gums you up. In addition, milk, and especially cheese contain lactose (milk sugar). Eight ounces of milk have approximately twelve grams of lactose that can break down into yeast, fungus - feeding sugars. If all that isn't enough, pasteurization (based on the fast germ theory) destroys any enzymes that might be there to begin with, and makes the milk "sick." Sick milk will rot and stink if left out, proving that pasteurization doesn't even work (can't kill microzymas), whereas raw milk will curdle naturally, and is still 'edible.' Last, but not least, dairy is highly acid-forming. This is all part of the immune storm attacking the body." (*Sick and Tired*, Dr. Young).

25. Question # Ani.25   What about coronary heart disease?

Coronary heart Disease (CHD) is the major cause of death in most Western countries. Serum total cholesterol concentration is the most important biochemical risk factor for CHD. Numerous studies have established that vegetarians have lower total serum cholesterol concentrations than comparable non-vegetarians. The relatively low serum total cholesterol of vegetarians has been observed in diverse populations, including white American Seventh-Day Adventists, American commune-dwelling vegans, American macrobiotic vegetarians, British vegetarians, elderly Chinese vegetarians, Slovakian vegetarians, West African Seventh-Day Adventists, Siberian vegans, German vegetarians, and many others. Furthermore, intervention trials have demonstrated that changing to a vegetarian diet can reduce serum cholesterol concentrations.

Vegetarian diets low in fat or saturated fat have been used successfully as part of comprehensive health programs to reverse severe coronary artery disease." (Journal of the

American Medical Association) In a study of more than 10,000 vegetarians and meat-eaters, British researchers found that the more meat consumed, the greater was the risk of heart attack.

"Vegetarian diets low in fat or saturated fat have been used successfully as part of comprehensive health programs to reverse severe coronary artery disease." Journal of the American Medical Association (1995)

Question # Ani.26 What about daily protein and bone loss?

The National Dairy Council keeps promoting that dairy products builds stronger bones but the research shows the contrary. "Osteoporosis is, in fact, a disease caused by a number of things, the most important of which is excess dietary protein! The correspondence between excess protein intake on bone resorption is direct and consistent, even with very high calcium intakes, the more excess protein in the diet the greater the incidence of negative calcium balance, and the greater the loss of calcium from the bones." (*Journal of Nutrition; American Journal of Clinical Nutrition; Journal of Bone and Joint Surgery*)

"One long-term study found that with as little as 75 grams of daily protein (less than three-quarters of what the average meat-eating American consumes) more calcium is lost in the urine than is absorbed by the body from the diet - a negative calcium balance. In every study the same correspondence was found: the more protein that is taken in, the more calcium that is lost. This is true even if the dietary calcium intake is as high as 1400 milligrams per day, far higher than the standard American diet." (*Protein and Calcium Loss a Review of the Nutrition Research; American Journal of Clinical Nutrition*)

"In other words, the more protein in our diet, the more calcium we lose, regardless of how much calcium we take in.

41

The result is that high-protein diets in general and meat-based diets in particular, lead to a gradual but inexorable decrease in bone density, and produce the ongoing development of osteoporosis." (*Journal of Nutrition*) This has been reported in numerous articles in the *Journal of Nutrition*.

27. Question # Ani.27   What about the acid vs. alkaline balance?

The average person on a meat-based diet eats two to three times the amount of protein that they actually need (80-120g for the average 150 lb. male). A plant-based diet provides the right amount of protein needed (35-54g for the average 150 lb. male) (35g is ideal and 54 is recommended for the average 150 lb. male.) The high protein level in an animal protein based diet causes acidosis. This acidosis starts because of the excess of uric acid that comes from the breakdown of excess amino acids in the body.

Distilled water is 7.0 pH and human milk is 7.43 pH which is the basis for man's normal pH. Thus our diet needs to be on the alkaline side of things to stay healthy. But the Standard American Diet is highly acidic and works off the 'extremes' found mostly in animal food and plant derivatives. Cooking is a form of food processing and is generally more acid forming. Raw foods are more alkalizing and cleansing for the body particularly after an extreme diet like the unhealthy Standard American Diet.

The homeostasis of the body seeks a 7.4 pH and other constant conditions such as a body temperature of 98.6 degrees F, certain glucose levels in the blood, certain amounts of body fluids etc. A major example of the importance of a balanced pH is given by Dr. Sherry Rogers, when she discusses how cancer cells become like yeast cells with a low pH (very acidic); "The normal pH of a cancer cell is 6.5, while a normal cell is 7.4. As soon as the pH of a cancer cell reaches 7.0, it stops growing; a little higher and it starts dying." "According to Cell Society, by Dr. S. Okada, cancer cells grow well in a culture solution produced by the metabolic wastes of regular cells. Since the metabolic waste material of regular cells is acidic, cancer cells, then, like this acidic condition."

A Dr. Theodore A. Baroody, N.D., D.C., Ph.D. points out, that: "Unfortunately, waste acids that are not eliminated when they should be are reabsorbed from the colon into the liver and put back into general circulation. They then deposit in the tissues. It is these tissue residues that determine sickness or health! Discover what tissue acid wastes are present and begin the process of alkalizing yourself, thus ridding them from the body. The result will be superior health, energy and strength to enjoy life fully. He further points out, "To replenish and sustain your alkaline reserves, follow the Rule of 80/20 – which means to eat 80% of your foods from the alkaline-forming list and 20% from the acid-forming list. Research, clinical experience, and the knowledge of the 'greats' in nutrition, have re-confirmed this ideal ratio of 80/20%."

Dr. Robert Young PhD. in his book, Sick and Tired Reclaim Your Inner Terrain, explains pH in the role of health and healing. "Most people today understand environmental pollution and how it sickens the Earth: we live off the planet and pollute it with waste. Well, illness is basically the same thing. These morbidly evolved organisms are literally eating us alive and polluting us. The thing is, we pollute ourselves first, thus creating the one physiological disease: pH imbalance/toxicity in our terrain. Toxins and an acid-forming diet disrupt body chemistry, and this loss of balance (i.e., dis-ease) in turn disturbs the central balance of the microzyma. Nutritional deficiencies can have the same effect, but can also be created by acidification: the evolution of microzymas is into bacteria and ultimately into a yeast and fungus Y/F infestation. Y/F can infest the blood and any cell or tissue, causing different symptoms.

"As more acid wastes back up and the body slowly stews in its own poisonous wastes, the acid begins to corrode veins, arteries, cells and tissues, leading to high valence cellular disorganization, which the medical community refers to as degenerative disease." "Normal body function and health require adequate alkaline reserves as well as the correct pH in tissues and blood. A major means of ensuring these conditions is the proper dietary ratio of alkaline to acid foods. A ratio of at least 80% to 20% - four parts alkaline to one part acid - is required (possibly 3 to 1 for a healthy person). When the proper ratio is maintained, morbid microforms are discouraged."

All animal products meat and dairy, are acidic and a lot of alkaline foods need to be eaten to keep a balanced pH. An unbalanced pH leads to degenerative diseases. The best choice is just to stay off of animal products.

28. Question # Ani.28   What about mutated and misformed meat-based Proteins?

This discussion crosses several areas of expertise and is complex. One raw food scholar David Wolfe, MS in chemistry, pointed out in his book, Eating for Beauty, that plant-based proteins have a single helix bond and meat-based proteins have a double helix bond. Also in the book, Genetic Roulette The Documented Health Risks of Genetically Engineered Foods (2007), and learned that genetic engineering is a huge multi-billion dollar business and it has a strong influence in the government. It also has become a world-wide health issue, with documented health-risks causing deaths, illnesses, diseases, and genetic engineering creates wide-spread, unpredictable changes in the food chain. This well researched book points out that: Proteins expressed in a Genetically Modified plant may be processed differently and those changes, which could include misfolding or molecular attachments, can be harmful in unpredicted ways. According to the Centre for Integrated Research on Biosafety

(INBI), 'proteins derived from natural sources generally regarded as safe can be [toxic to cells] if allowed to re-fold under different conditions.' Sometimes, refolding can result in groups of proteins aggregating into shapes with harmful consequences. INBI points out that certain aggregations of "proteins that have sustained mutations or have been misfolded" (amyloid fibrils) are involved in a variety of medical conditions such as Alzheimer's and Parkinson's diseases.'" (Nature)

Furthermore, the mitochondrial damage is a known issue with Parkinson's. A little known fact is that meat-based protein is different on the molecular level than plant-based protein. Meat-based protein has a double-helix bond whereas plant-based protein has a single-helix bond, making it more flexible, and it takes less energy to break down in the ATP cycle. Research into Parkinson's disease finds that: 'Mutated and misformed proteins tend to aggregate.' (J Biol Chem) The Lewy bodies in the brains of Parkinson's patients, the neurological problems in the brains of MS and the high levels of amyloid plaque found in Alzheimer's in the brain are also directly related to high animal protein levels in the body. Explaining a little of the details will help. The Embden-Meyerhof glycolytic pathway and the Krebs' Cycle both have as their starting point protein which breaks down to amino acids (and to glucose and ketones). This is the final pathway that all nutrient metabolites are involved in for energy production which involves the mitochondria. The studies on Parkinson's have found that: 'The concept that mitochondrial dysfunction can cause a Parkinsonian syndrome came into focus with the observation that MPTP induced PD in drug addicts. (Psychiatry Res; Science) Mitochondrial dysfunctions are now recognized to be the major cause of nigral degeneration in experimental models of PD and possibly even in idiopathic PD (J Neurochem; Bioessays).

So in other words, meat-based proteins, which are amino acids that have a double-helix bond, are considered abnormal proteins. Whereas, plant-based proteins which are single-helix bonds, are considered the ideal type of proteins for humans. This buildup of animal-based proteins not only causes inflammation, it also causes the growth of fungi and causes a buildup of excess protein-based substances that eventually could end up in the Lewy bodies and amyloid plaque found in the brain of MS, Parkinson's and Alzheimer's. The Lewy Bodies and other deformed proteins in the brains of PD, MS and Alzheimer's patients are animal-based proteins (double helix bonds) which are dead foods or misformed proteins and this could also be from genetic engineering. Plant-based proteins (single helix bonds) which are Living Foods do not mutate or become misformed proteins that aggregate. Live-Food diets have cured both PD and MS, (also for Alzheimer's and ALS there is some evidence of cures) by replacing the misformed or distorted proteins with healthy plant-based proteins. In MRI's the brain scar tissue also has been shown to clear up as part of the process of eating a raw vegan diet.

In addition, the pathogenic microorganisms that enter the body through meat-based diets end up in the gut and the liver and can end up in the brain, which is one of the reasons why there is protein aggregation in the brain such as with Lewy bodies. This is all a technical discussion but it gives a basic understanding of the mutated and misformed meat-based proteins.

29. Question #Ani.29   What about the China Study on Animal Protein?

The retired professor emeritus of Nutritional Sciences, at Cornell University, Colin Campbell PhD, has a chapter on Osteoporosis in his nationally known book: The China Study, (2005) The world famous "China Study" was the longest and largest nutrition study ever done. "Americans consume more cow's milk and its products per person than most populations in the world. So Americans should have wonderfully strong bones, right? Unfortunately not. A recent study showed that American women aged fifty and older have one of the highest rates of hip fractures in the world. (J. Gerontology) The only countries with higher rates are in Europe and in the south Pacific (Australia and New Zealand) (J. Gerontology) where they consume even more milk than the United States.

Furthermore, Dr. Campbell adds: "when women in America, such as those in the Nurses' Health Study (Cancer Epi. Biom. Prev.) and the billion-dollar Women's Health Trial, (J. Natl. Cancer Inst.; Prev. Med.; Controlled Clin. Trials) reduce their fat intake, they do not do it by reducing their consumption of animal-based foods. Instead, they use low-fat and nonfat animal products, along with less fat during cooking and at the table. Thus, they are not adopting the diets that were shown, in the international correlation studies and in our rural China study, to be associated with low breast cancer rates. This is a very important discrepancy, and is illustrated by the correlation between the consumption of dietary animal protein and dietary fat for a group of countries. (*Am. Journ. Clin. Nutr.; Int. J. Cancer; Cancer Epi. Biom. Prev.*) The most reliable comparison was published in 1975; (Int. J. Cancer) it showed a highly convincing correlation of more than 90%. This means that as fat intake goes up in various countries, animal protein intake increases in an almost perfectly parallel manner. Likewise, in the China Study, the intakes of fat and animal protein also show a similar correlation of 84%." (Diet, life-style and mortality in the *China Study*. A study of the characteristics of 65 Chinese counties. Oxford, UK; Ithaca, NY)

Dr. Campbell further notes: "When animal protein increases metabolic acid and draws calcium from the bones, the amount of calcium in the urine is increased. This effect has been established for over eighty years and has been studied in some detail since the 1970's. Summaries of these studies were published in 1974, (*Am. J. Clin. Nutr.*) 1981 (*J. Nutr.*) and 1990. (*J. Nutr.*) Each of these summaries clearly shows that the amount of animal protein consumed by many of us on a daily basis is capable of causing substantial increases in urinary calcium. Doubling protein intake (mostly animal-based) from 35-78 g/day causes an alarming 50% increase in urinary calcium. (*J. Nutr.*) This effect occurs well within the range of protein intake that most of us consume; average American intake is around 70-100 g/day. Incidentally, a six-month study funded by the Atkins Center found that those people who adopted the Atkins Diet excreted 50% more calcium in their urine after six months on the diet." (*Am J. Med.*)

"T. Colin Campbell, a Professor of Nutritional Sciences at Cornell University and the senior science advisor to the American Institute for Cancer Research, says there is 'a strong correlation between dietary protein intake and cancer of the breast, prostate, pancreas and colon. The culprit in many of the most prevalent and deadly diseases of our time, according to this study, is none other than the very thing many of us have been taught to hold virtually sacred - animal protein. People who derive 70% of their protein from animal products have major health difficulties compared to people who derive just 5% of their protein from animal sources. They have 17 times the death rate from heart disease and the women are 5 times more likely to die of breast cancer. In conclusion, animal protein is at the core of many chronic diseases." (Young, Robert, and Young, Shelly, *Back to the House of Health, and Back to the House of Health II*).

30. Question #Ani.30 What about the Paleo Diet?

The Paleo Diet is close to a raw vegan or Live-Food diet except for the inclusion of meat. This diet mimics the diets of the hunter-gatherer ancestors with common everyday foods. Loren Cordain the creator of the diet states: "It is not crucial to exactly duplicate hunter-gather diets. This would be a next-to-impossible tasks in our twenty-first-century

world, as many of those foods are no longer in existence, are commercially unavailable, or are simply unpalatable to our contemporary tastes and cultural biases." (*The Paleo Diet revised*, Loren Cordain, PhD)

One of the best analyses of the Paleo Diet is the nationally known author, speaker on plant-based diets and registered dietitian, Brenda Davis, RD, see her website.

The first major mistake he makes is that hunter-gathers did not eat supermarket foods but ate wild organic fruits, vegetables and grasses which according to David Wolf citing the literature, a raw food expert, are 10 to 20 times more nutritious.

His second basic mistake is he says you can eat all the lean meats, poultry, fish, seafoods you can consume. But studies of ancient people like the Jews in biblical times indicate they ate meat about once a week, or as one doctoral dissertation concluded 3 times a month. The Romans and wealthy who ate meat daily had the same degenerative diseases as today. And eating all the meat you want brings up the issues in questions 11 thru 29 mentioned here. Eating meat on a daily basis is definitely a bad thing as noted in the review of the literature mentioned in questions 11 through 29 for dangers and 1 through 42 for other reasons.

Third hunter-gathers ate raw meat, probably within an hour or so after killing the animal. Within an hour after an animal is killed its biochemistry starts to change to acidic and other negative properties (parasites, yeast, mold, fungus) which start to set in, even if frozen.

All the problems and dangers of a meat-based diet in questions 11 through 29 can be applied to the Paleo meat-based diet; it is no different than any other meat-based diet, especially if they are eating red meat and meat on a daily basis. Things already discussed like antibiotics, pathogenic

microorganisms, bone loss, protein clogging the base membranes, heavy metal toxicity, and acidic levels will be high and other issues already discussed in ques. 11-29. Loren Cordain understands the problems with grains, dairy products, refined sugars, and processed foods but doesn't seem to understand all the problems with meat and does not mention them!

All meat-based diets, no matter what the rest of the diet involves, they have the same problem and dangers mentioned in questions 11 through 29.

The thing that is different in the Paleo diet from other meat-based diets is that it cuts out: grains, dairy products, refined sugars, and processed foods and the emphasis to stick to this 85% or more of the time. That is a start in the right direction, but eating meat at every meal, especially the emphasis on red meat, should be reduced to no more than three times a week, that animal protein would be allowed. The reason for mentioning the Paleo is that it is a better option than most meat-based diets because of all it cuts out. Yet a Live-Food diet is still more advanced and healthier.

Fred Bisci, PhD a clinical nutritionists and nationally known raw fooder of over 40 years has a book, Your Healthy Journey, that is helpful here. He has an option for his intermediate eating lifestyle for those who feel they need meat. He only recommends eating fish, chicken and turkey and no more than three times a week every other day. His next stage of the advanced eating lifestyle eliminates animal products completely. This is especially true for those with degenerative diseases. His website: www.fredbisci4health.com

Even though the Paleo diet has some good suggestions, if you want to eat meat get Fred Bisci, PhD's book, *Your Healthy Journey* and follow his suggestion for a meat-based diet.

Eating a small amount of meat only three times a week, every other day is a very good suggestion.

Dr. Robert Young points out: "Eating meat can give us protein; however, along with this protein comes saturated fat and possible synthetic hormones, steroids, and antibiotics have been given to the animal. Also, pesticide chemicals can be in the meat from the grain fed to the animal to fatten it up. Along with all of this, morbid pathogenic bacteria loads from the fermentation of acids can be present in the animal tissues, before or at the time of slaughter."

Many people are under the assumption that poultry is a completely different type of meat then beef, but not really. When it dies it goes through the same postmortem changes. The biophysical and biochemical changes that poultry muscle undergoes postmortem are, in general, the same as those reported for various mammalian species. The most apparent change, of course, is the stiffening of muscle as it passes into rigor mortis. The chemical changes that accompany this physical change are: 1) Disappearance of ATP; 2) the appearance of ammonia and inosinic acid; 3) the accumulation of lactic acid (This lowers the pH from above 7.0 to ultimate values of 5.7 to 5.9.). In red meats postmortem changes in pH vary according to the type of red meat, both the rate of pH decline and the depth of decline vary from a slow gradual decline in 24 hours to a rapid decline of 30 to 90 minutes. The pH falls from about 6.7 and 7.0 to 5.0 to 6.0. The paler the meat the more the pH drops. The color changes from a darker to a pale meat and the muscle stiffens. As the pH is declining the proteins denature. The muscle of fish is different from that of mammals and birds. "The lowest postmortem pH which is reached in many species of food fish is in the range of about 6.2 to 6.6; but in some species, such as halibut, tuna, mackerel, and shark, it many fall to between 5.5 to 6.0."

31. Question #Ani.31   What about the Kosher Diet?

A fascinating study by a researcher, Dr. David Macht of Johns Hopkins University, looked at Leviticus XI and Deuteronomy XIV. He did a study in which he reported the toxic effects of animal flesh on a controlled growth culture. A substance was classified as toxic if it slowed the culture's growth rate below 75 percent. In each case, the blood, of all the animals Dr. Macht tested showed up more toxic than the flesh." (Bulletin of Historical Medicine, Johns Hopkins University)

His results show that the lower the growth percentage of the culture, the more toxic the flesh. Note that the flesh of animals and fish given to us by God for food are all nontoxic, but all forbidden animals lie in the toxic range.

Here we find that science has confirmed the Bible's list of clean versus unclean animals! Apparently the Jews understood the biochemistry of toxicity 3,500 years ago, or perhaps God knew this and was warning the Jews for their health and safety! And the animals that are 'clean' are those that are vegetarians! It is the meat-eaters and scavengers (pigs, shrimp, and lobsters) that eat anything and everything that are unclean.

Basic science would indicate that animals that eat other animals would have higher toxic percentage then animals that ate leaves and grass. Animals store toxins and poisons in their fat cells and the more animals other animals eat the higher the toxin and poisons rate in their cells. The Jews were in line with basic biochemistry and toxicology!

This scientist was basically comparing those animals classified as kosher to those animals classified as non-kosher in the Bible. All those animals that are kosher or nontoxic were in the safe range for human consumption with low toxicity levels. But the non-kosher animals all had high toxicity levels that would be considered unsafe for human consumption. In other words, all forbidden animals in the bible lie in the toxic range. As it turned out the toxic animals are all meat eaters, while the non-toxic animals are vegetarians! This confirmed the biblical insight concerning meat consumption, when the people rebelled and wanted to eat meat.' God wants people to eat a pure diet and when a person has a disease they need to go through a process of physiological purification to get the body back to its pure, natural, complete state of health and life.

32. Question # Ani.32   What is a list of some dangers of excess protein?

1. Surplus protein ends up being stored as fat. Both meat and cheese have much more fat then protein in them.
2. Animal protein usually contains excess fat and excess cholesterol, these increase the risk of chronic diseases such as: arthritis, diabetes, cancer.
3. "According to a report by the National Research Council, fat is not the only thing that promotes tumor growth. At the very least, the cancer-stimulating effects of excess fat and protein may turn out to reinforce each other." (Food and Nutrition Board) Moreover, the extra ammonia that results from the breakdown of excess protein has even been thought to hasten cell proliferation and to contribute to the development of malignant growths." (American Journal of Clinical Nutrition)
4. "Researchers (Journal of American College of Nutrition) have shown that even purified animal protein, devoid of cholesterol, when substituted for vegetable protein, is associated with a significant rise in serum cholesterol."
5. Protein breaks down into ammonia and urea both of which are possible toxic nitrogen by-products. Ammonia is carcinogenic and urea promotes arthritis. "Dr. C. L. Elvehjem in 'Amino Acid Supplementation of Cereal' warns that twice the daily requirement of certain amino acids in food leads to toxic cell disturbance. Dr. Bieler states that one of the main sources of over acidity in the body is an excess of amino acids which disturbs the nitrogen balance."
6. The sulfur by-product needs alkaline reserves to neutralize

it, yet most people's Standard American meat-based diets, are acidic.

7. Bone minerals, calcium and magnesium are used to neutralize sulfur causing a loss of these bone minerals, and possibly causing osteoporosis. (Journal of Bone and Joint Surgery)

"Throughout the world, the incidence of osteoporosis correlates directly with protein intake. In any given population, the greater the intake of protein, the more common and more severe will be the osteoporosis. In fact, the world health statistics show that osteoporosis is most common in exactly those countries where dairy products are consumed in the largest quantities - the United States, Finland, Sweden, and the United Kingdom." (American Journal of Clinical Nutrition)

8. "One study showed that even a daily 2,300-milligram supplement of calcium could not compensate for the mineral-robbing effects of excess protein, and many other studies have documented the adverse effects of excessive protein intake on calcium loss as well. (American Journal of Clinical Nutrition; Journal of Nutrition)

9. Amyloid deposits cause degenerative changes, a shorter lifespan and premature aging from excess protein.

10. Cooking meat creates mutagens which alters the DNA of a cell increasing the risk of cancer and other degenerative diseases.

11. Research suggests that excess protein can be damaging to the kidneys and that high-protein diets may well contribute to the decline in kidney function that occurs as one grows older, usually this is attributed to old age. "It is important to recall that current experiments suggest that excess protein can be damaging to the kidneys. (New England Journal of Medicine) Researchers also feel that high-protein diets may well contribute to the decline in kidney function that occurs as one grows older and that has been attributed to normal aging.

12. Other studies suggest that diets high in animal protein increase one's risk of kidney stones and gallstones. (Clinical Science)

13. The world's food reserves are used up faster by those

who eat excess protein since meat protein takes far more food reserves then does vegetable proteins. A person can live on one acre of soy protein but it takes 8 acres to live off of meat. 14. Meat stirs up lust, anger, greed and other negative passions of the soul, which increases violence, rape and murder. Monastics referred to the negative passions of the soul concerning meat eating and thus many were vegetarians.

Plant-based Health and History
(His. is history questions)

33. Question #His.33   What about vegetarian detoxification and health?

To have a superior healthy vegetarian dietary lifestyle has two parts: Diet and Detox. This two-fold system is necessary for a person to attain Superior Health. It is one thing to take the right foods in but it is also necessary to detox and get the wastes and poisons and toxins out of the body too. In a way diet and exercise is learning to manage your personal energy. As we move along we learn to use whatever is needed to get the maximum energy needed for our life. Whereas half the battle is getting the nutrients in the other half is the detox and getting out what should come out.

Detox means detoxification and also the detoxification system. The natural way everybody detoxifies is through defecation and urination, sweating and sneezing, etc. But because of our diet and other things these natural ways are not enough anymore. But there are other ways and here are some of the other commonly used methods of detoxification.

1. Exercise and Aerobics.
2. On a daily basis drink lots of water.
3. Fasting (once a week and a yearly long fast)
4. Enemas and Colonics.
5. Sauna's and hot baths.
6. Massage, Dry Skin Brush Massage and Reflexology.

7. Polarity Therapy, Acupuncture...
8. Herbs and Supplements that detox.
9. Living Food diets can be helpful in detox.

There is a little known system in the body called the detoxification system. We have many different systems in the body: the respiratory system; the cardiovascular system; the gastrointestinal system; the musculoskeletal system; the endocrine system; the nervous system; the immune system; and the detoxification system. This is a biochemical system used to clean out toxins in the body. But in order for the detoxification system and most other body systems to work properly the right amount and kind of nutrients are needed.

34. Question #His.34   What is the Ideal or Perfect diet for humans?

The ideal diet is found in the Garden of Eden, but we cannot go back to there so we accommodate and get close to it which is 100% Living Foods. The ideal diet would be the 100% Raw Living Foods Vegan Lifestyle, with organic produce. But this ideal could be difficult to achieve for some and for others a transition period may be needed, and others may have a hard time obtaining organic produce. In addition the consensus of the Living Foods community varies as to the exact nature of a raw living foods lifestyle. Some emphasis only 100% raw others, 95%, others 80/20. Some emphasize no grains others limited use of grains.
Some emphasize only organic others it doesn't matter that much. Some exclude certain foods, others use all types of foods. Some exclude any use of supplements others encourage it. But the Living Foods community consensus is much closer and better defined then the medical and academic community on diet.

Consensus in the medical and academic community takes a long time. It took 30 years to prove that high cholesterol levels cause heart disease. A more reasonable holistic approach is to consider the animal and cell culture studies data as preliminary since some of these are controversial and could be wrong (ex. Shark cartilage to reduce cancer). When there's a majority of clinical studies present then there is a very good chance it is true. Good science should be based mostly on clinical studies. For over 40 years studies (scientific, cross-cultural and historical) have been done on vegetarians and have proven time and time again that a vegetarian diet is healthier, yet the majority of the medical and academic community does not listen.

35. Question #His.35   What about the different dietary schools of thought?

Most every book that you pick up on health food emphasizes that there are some foods that are good for you and some foods are not very good for you. Or perhaps it would be better stated, some foods and diets are very good, some are just O.K. and some are very poor for individuals. Most of these books try to move people away from eating meat and fat, processed and cooked foods, to a more vegetarian diet. There is some real truth in these facts and beliefs.

Different cultures require different dietary patterns for their country. Moreover each individual has slightly different physiological needs, genetically. Even seasonal changes; fall, winter, spring, and summer have different demands on the human body and would require a different dietary need. On top of this is the need for individual healing that may require a certain dietary orientation for a while. Thus there is not one diet that is the perfect diet, individually or globally. As an old saying goes, one shoe does not fit all. But some are better than others.

There are dozens of schools of thought and many books have been written on these. Most of them can be put into categories or clusters of theories and practices. We are not interested in the many meat-based diet schools of thought, for reasons stated. Raw food cuisine has shunned the stigma of "health food" and is becoming known as a new exciting food group that is actually superior to health foods. And it brings superior health, beyond what the standard American diet or even health food diets can bring. And there are well known professionals in the field that give the movement validity and a solid foundation.

A distinction needs to be made from the Whole Living Foods Vegan movement and the vegetarian movement that has been around for many years in many different ways. These are two different dietary lifestyles or clusters. Most of these vegetarian diets out today would fall more into the Health Food Diet cluster but some of the stricter vegetarians and the vegans could be considered the Raw Vegan or Living Foods Diet cluster.

I would hypothesize that there seems to be three basic clusters of dietary health, one on top of the other. Within each circle are numerous smaller groups of the various Nutritional Schools of Thought and Theories. Like a snowman with three balls of snow one bigger at the bottom a smaller in the middle and a small head at the top.

The first, highest and healthiest cluster of dietary theories are the Vegan and Raw Vegan Diets which has a very small following, it is not easy living in the world today to live up to those standards. By Raw I mean Raw Living Foods, a little to no cooking, at least 80/20 or above (80% raw, 20% or less cooked or processed. Raw live fruits and vegetables are the basis.

The second cluster is the Health Food Diets cluster which is growing bigger and used by most people in the preventative health field today. This is a mixed bag and is composed of numerous health food oriented diets and practices and schools of thought. What puts them in this category is that they all have different variations of cooked and processed foods with an emphasis on grains as the basis.

The third and largest cluster is the Standard American Diets (SAD) cluster which is where most people are involved today, unfortunately it is a diet of slow suicide through poisons and toxins in foods. This is the standard meat and potatoes, with milk and cookies diet of the U.S. population. The SAD diet is the Standard American Degenerative Diet.

There is a natural tendency in our bodies to evolve but this takes time. The important thing is to start moving your diet from the Standard American Diet to a Health Food Diet that would be a great accomplishment in and of itself. Then follow your Heart and move into the Raw Food movement and Living Foods. A Raw or Live-Foods diet is superior and optimal to other dietary lifestyles; it is the best diet and brings the most health and longest life.

36. Question # His.36   Is there a historical progression of health movements?

Yes, there is a historical progression. The history of clinical nutrition can be divided into four distinct eras: the first began in the nineteenth century and extended into the early twentieth century when it was recognized for the first time that food contained constituents which were essential for human function and that different foods provided different amounts of these essential agents.

The second era was initiated in the early decades of the twentieth century and might be called "the vitamin period." Vitamins came to be recognized in foods and deficiency syndromes were described. In the third era of nutritional history in the early 1950's to mid-1960's, vitamin therapy began to fall into disrepute. Concomitants with this, nutrition

education in medical schools also became less popular.

As this educational vacuum developed, due to the reduced emphasis on nutrition in medical institutions, it was filled by lay nutritionists and individuals who purported to have miracle cures using nutritional remedies. As a result, in the 60's and 70's have seen a reputation surrounding nutrition grow as a "soft science" with little relevance to clinical medicine as long as a person is consuming foods from the four food groups.

Due to the recognition of the relationship of disease to the malnutrition of overconsumption/ under-nutrition, there has been a winning back of the sympathies of many health practitioners as to the importance of nutrition in terms of reflection upon the total diet and the impact of diet on specific individuals in the prevention of nutrient-related syndromes. This signals the fourth period of nutrition evolution in the early 1980's, which has witnessed the reintroduction of nutrition courses within the curricula of many schools training health practitioners and a new heightened emphasis on nutritional biochemistry and the role that nutrition can play in a total preventive health-care program. Raw vegan and Living Foods started in the 70's and 80's.

Now a fifth era of nutrition has opened up in the 1990's in the area of the Raw, Living Foods Vegan movement, not only in terms of personal health but also in terms of clinical application. It is the highest and most optimal form of dietary lifestyle. Raw Living Foods have been around since the time of Adam and Eve in the Garden and people though-out history have eaten this way. But in the last twenty to thirty years (1980's to 2013) this era of nutrition has matured both in science and in the practice of the Live-Foods culinary arts.

37. Question # His.37 Is religion a factor with plant-based diets?

Most of the major religious leaders were vegetarian or close to it. See Jim Tibbetts book: *Jesus and Mary were Kosher Vegetarians, the evidence from the Bible, the early Church and Nutrition.*

One researcher noted: "Those people who are observant of a religious faith (regardless of which particular sect or denomination) enjoy lower incidence and mortality than the general population. Regular attendance at church services has been associated with lowered mortality from several chronic diseases. The possibility that some aspect of spiritual life or some other lifestyle highly correlated with spirituality explains the lower cancer risk in religious denominations that espouse vegetarianism must be considered."

The Seventh Day Adventists are a group that has been studied because of their beliefs and diets. In a medical journal, Dr. Jeremiah Stamler, a cardiologist was talking about lifestyles and demonstrated with statistics on death rate quotes. He noted that: "An additional comparison has recently become available, with data on mortality for three groups of California Seventh Day Adventists (non-vegetarian, lacto-ovo-vegetarian and pure vegetarian) compared with the California general population. Seventh Day Adventists have lower mean serum cholesterol levels than Americans generally. For 47,000 Seventh Day Adventist men (aged 35 and over, age-sex-standardized) mortality rates were 34% lower for non-vegetarians, 57% lower for the lacto-ovo-vegetarians and 77% lower for the pure vegetarians compared to the general population. The results were evident that the strict dietary standards of the Adventists made them much healthier. The Adventist men had a heart attack mortality rate only 12 percent that of the average California male. Lung cancer was reduced 80 percent; uterine cancer in women was reduced 46 percent. In nearly every major disease, Adventists ranked well below the average in risk. And they lived an average of ten years longer than the average Californian.

Protection to the Environment
   (Environment is Env.)

Question #Env.38   Is animal protein a problem for the environment?

Bal tashchit, is a Jewish law or tenet which means to give protection to the environment. Protection of the environment (bal tashchit) means that the earth is the Lord's and the people are partners and co-workers with God in protecting the environment. "The earth is the Lord's and the fullness thereof." Ps 24:1

Another 'bal taschit' definition is that it means, Conservation of Resources. Waste or unnecessary destruction is prohibited as given in Deuteronomy 20:19-20,
which prohibits the destruction of fruit bearing trees (in time of warfare).

Global Warming has three main causes:
Automobiles, Industry and Cattle!

Pollution and CO_2 from cars and industry is well understood but the third reason cattle and the meat-based diet needs some explanation. Feeding massive amounts of grain and water to animals on factory farms, trucking the animals around slaughtering them, and refrigerating their bodies so that they don't rot wastes a ton of energy. In fact, producing 1 calorie of meat uses more than 10 times the amount of fossil fuel that it takes to produce 1 calorie of plant foods, like beans, veggies, and grains. Some of the main problems with the environment which are either directly or indirectly related to a meat-based diet are as follows.

A person can live on one acre of soybeans but it takes 8 acres for a person to live off of animal products. Figuring the fossil fuels in concerning animal production and sales it takes upwards of 15 times over plant-based fossil fuel productions.

39. Question # Env.39 What does the United Nations say about animal foods?

According to the United Nations, raising animals for food is 'one of the top two or three most significant contributors to the most serious environmental problems, at every scale from local to global.

On C-Span (4/2012) there was a conference on; "Global Renewable and Sustainable Energy Development," by the Center for Global Development. A number of professionals in this field spoke including the United Nations Secretary General: Ban-Ki-Moon. He explained that today "we are using 1.3 times the earth's resources that we have." "If we continue this way, it's like we have 5 planet earths, what we are doing is acting as if there is no tomorrow." "The leaders are most important, it is important to have leaders commit themselves to change."

He stated that he was speaking to finance ministers from around the world and stated that, "challenges are of such immense magnitude that it requires nothing more than paradigm shifts, in order to achieve a green economy." "We have to change our behavior patterns since we have limited resources." He explained that we are heading towards a tipping point (for the worst) in climate change. Of the different issues he listed one was the food crisis another was water resources. "The power of partnership is needed for this endeavor." He and others spoke at this event.

40. Question # Env.40 What about land and water usage concerning meat?

One source stated that a person can live on one acre of

soybeans for a whole year, but for a cow it takes 8 acres of land to provide protein for one person for a year; this is a 8 to 1 ratio. Another source cited below gives a 12 to 1 ratio. Even though there is a debate in the math, it is at least 8 to 1.

"There is only about one acre of agricultural land on this earth, per person, at the present population level. One fourth of an acre or less is needed to feed a person if he lives on a vegetarian diet. But three acres or more are needed if he depends on animal protein for food. (a) While one acre will produce, as beef 77 days' worth of protein for a man, the same acre would produce 236 days of protein in milk, 877 days in whole wheat, or 2,224 days in soybeans. (b)"

"A beef animal must consume one hundred calories to produce ten calories in meat. It takes twenty-one pounds of protein fed to cattle to get one pound of protein in return. Pigs and chickens do a little better, but averaging all classes of food animals, eight pounds of protein in feed are required to get one pound of protein in return."

Animal agriculture uses 70 percent of the world's agricultural land and 30 percent of the planet's total land area.

Water Usage
"Another matter: More and more, water is being recognized as a resource in short supply. An all-vegetarian regimen requires 300 gallons of water daily for each person. A mixed animal and vegetable diet requires 2,500 gallons daily per person. The cost of water per pound is 25 times that of the cost per pound of vegetarian food."

41. Question # Env.41 What about medical expenses and animal consumption?

Medical costs are indirectly related to the environment. The annual medical costs in the United States directly attributable to smoking: $65 billion. The annual medical costs in the

United States directly attributable to meat consumption: $60-120 billion. This figure greatly increases if the costs of degenerative diseases is added since a lot of evidence shows a meat-based diet is a primary cause or one of the causes of diseases like heart disease.

42. Question # Env.42   What about CO2 pollution increasing and animals?

Methane is a 'greenhouse gas' which traps about 25 times as much solar heat as CO2. Annually the world's 1.3 billion cows produce about 100 million tons of methane.

The U.S. lost 70 million acres of forest land during 70 years last century, over two thirds of it to grazing land. In Latin America, the demand for cattle grazing land is the cause of the ongoing destruction of the tropical rain forest. About a 1000 acres a year are lost in Latin America. All of this caused increased CO2 and reduced Oxygen levels.

The greenhouse effect of the destruction of the ozone layer is caused in large part by pollution from cattle. "Loss of forest land in the United States is a serious problem, rapidly getting worse. In 1900, there were about 509 million acres of non-federal forest land in the United States, but by 1950 this had declined to 420 million acres, and in 1975 it had declined further to 376 million acres. (a) Analysis of use conversion between 1967 and 1975 reveals that most conversions of forest land were to grazing land. We lost 70 million acres of forest land during this time, over two thirds of it to grazing land. (b)" "What is the cause of the ongoing destruction of tropical forest? In Latin America, the demand for cattle grazing land is probably the dominant factor."

"Every nation's relative contribution to global warming includes the United States (30.3%); which is responsible for more greenhouse gas pollution than South America (3.8%); Africa (2.5%); the middle East (2.6%), Australia (1.1%);

Japan (3.7%); and Asia, India, China (12.2%), all put together. All of Europe (27.7%); Russia (13.7%) and Canada (2.3%)."

"In another example on the carbon emissions per person, the world average is 1 ton of carbon per person, whereas for the U.S. it is 5.5 tons of carbon per person. In another example; "At no point in the last 650,000 years before the pre-industrial era did the CO_2 concentration go above 300 parts per million." Now it is about 375 and in 45 years it'll be above 600.

The fall of 2011 the world's population reached 7 billion people, the increase in population has decreased the amount of oxygen in the air and increased the amount of CO_2 in the air. Both the loss of vegetation and the increase in human population has caused the increase in CO_2. About 4% of the human race who live in the United States produce about 25% of the carbon dioxide. About 40% of global warming is the U.S. responsibility.

Measurements of oxygen trapped in rocks about ten thousands of years ago showed that the earth had about 39% oxygen in the air back then. Today the amount of oxygen in the air is about 18 to 20%.

In January of 2008 a leading climatologist, Jim Hansen at NASA, and his team published a paper saying that they looked at all the paleoclimate data and they looked at the observational data from the last few years and finally were able to say: "any value of carbon in the atmosphere greater than 350 parts per million is not compatible with the planet on which civilization developed and to which life on the earth is adapted." As noted above the CO_2 level in 2006 was 375 parts per million and it is rising about 2 parts per million per year.

Bill McKibben an author in this area writes in an article, "What It Will Take to Return the Globe to 350" that in 2010 the world was 390 parts per million. "We are already way past where we should be. [350] That is why the arctic is melting. That is why the ocean is 30 percent more acid than it used to be, and why it is beginning to unravel the marine food chain. It is why all of these things are going on. It is why we are really in the process of de-creating the planet in a very powerful ways. So that is the bad news.

"The scientists' proclamation about 350 parts per million was the good news to us as organizers because the two things that translate across the world's frustrating linguistic boundaries are musical notation and Arabic numbers. Having this number, 350, meant that we could try to build a global campaign. ..."

43. Question # Env.43 What about the increasing population and food production?

"Increasing food production on a global scale is a problem of critical importance and it is exacerbated further by the addition of 200,000 persons per day in the world population. However, the increasing world's need for food is due, not only to the growing population, but also to rising affluence. In some developing countries, the average person is sustained by the equivalent of about 400 lb of cereal per year, consumed directly, whereas in the United States, per capita requirement for cereal grain is nearly 2000 lb, most of it fed to animals and consumed ultimately as meat, eggs, and dairy products. It has been estimated that 91% of the cereal, legume, and vegetable protein produced in the United States, and suitable for human use, is fed to livestock."

"While the rich are dying from diseases of affluence, the poor of the planet languish from want of the bare essentials of life. The injustice imposed on the world by the twentieth-century protein chain is unprecedented; a billion people gorging and purging, mired in excess fat, while a billion more waste away, unable to provide their bodies with the minimum nutrient requirements necessary to maintain a healthy existence. The World Bank estimates that between 700 million and 1 billion people live in absolute poverty around the world. Contrary to popular belief, the poor are getting poorer each year. Forty-three developing nations finished the 1980's poorer than they were at the beginning of the decade. Approximately 20 million people die each year around the world from hunger and related diseases. Over 15 million children die every year from diseases brought on by or complicated by malnutrition."

"A Harvard nutritionist, Jean Mayer, estimates that reducing meat production by just 10% would release enough grain to feed 60 million people. The shocking and tragic truth is that 80-90% of all grain grown in America is used to feed meat animals." Another work also states, "In this country one half of our harvested agricultural land is planted with feed crops. In fact, we feed 78 percent of all our grain to animals. The high quality food we feed to livestock is wasted. Cattle, sheep, and goats do not need to eat protein in order to produce protein."

About the year 1800 there were 1 billion people. Between 1930 and 1999 the world grew from 2 billion to 6 billion. Between 2000 and 2011 the world grew to 7 billion. Thus in 70 years the world grew by 4 billion and in the last 10 years it grew another 1 billion people. In 30-40 years we could reach 10 billion people.

Back in the 1980's China's scientists did the math and realized that their country, which now has a billion people, could only support so many people with their limited land mass. So they instituted the one child policy per family. The world's population is now at 7 billion people and estimates show that around 10 billion people is the limit since the earth's resources cannot support that large number of people for a long time.

The carbon footprint of a meat-based diet is huge, much

bigger than a plant-based diet. Now with 7 billion people, the world needs to go back to its vegetarian roots.

44. Question # Env.44 What about increasing temperatures, sea levels and hurricanes?

As noted previously cattle and animal food production is affecting the climate and fossil fuel usage, water, land and other issues. These then in term affect increasing temperatures, sea levels and hurricanes.

The earth's mean temperature has not varied more than 3.6 degrees Fahrenheit since the last Ice Age, 18,000 years ago. Many scientists now predict a 4- to 9-degree rise in the earth's surface temperature over the next fifty years as we continue to spew carbon dioxide, methane, nitrous oxide, and chloroflurocarbons into the atmosphere, blocking solar heat from escaping the planet.

A temperature change of this magnitude is likely to plunge the world's ecosystems and human civilization into the throes of an unprecedented crisis. Again the increased temperatures caused by Global Warming are directly connected to the meat-based diet.

NASA said that 2010 had the warmest twelve months on record. The first three months of 2012 are clearly the warmest months in U.S. history, it will probably beat 2010.

Scientists predict a three- to five- foot rise in seawater level by the year 2050 as a result of thermal heat expansion of the oceans. If the polar icecaps melt, the rise in water level would be even higher and whole landmasses will disappear from the face of the earth.

The Environmental Protection Agency predicts that a five-foot rise in sea level would destroy up to 90 percent of America's remaining wetlands.

"On July 31, 2005, less than a month before Hurricane Katrina hit the United States, a major study from MIT supported the scientific consensus that global warming is making hurricanes more powerful and more destructive. Major storms spinning in both the Atlantic and the Pacific since the 1970's have increased in duration and intensity by about 50%. The cost: Great Weather and Flood Catastrophes, Losses in Billions of U.S. dollars: 1960-1969 about 25 billion; 1980-1989 about 50 billion; 1988-1997 about 275 billion; 1998-2005 about 675 billion.

In 2011 and 2012 in the U.S. there is some concern the number of increasing tornados over previous years and also about their increased level of intensity.

45. Question # Env.45 What is an Environmentally Conscious Eating approach?

An Environmentally Conscious Eating approach is understanding diet from the perspective of its impact on the topsoil, water supplies, air, animal population, human population, and its effect on peace in the world and avoidance of sins!

Former Vice President Al Gore outlines the major problem of Global Warming in his book (2006), An Inconvenient Truth. Al Gore opened the book: "We have everything we need to begin solving this crisis, with the possible exception of the will to act. But in America, our will to take action is itself a renewable resource." "And those with the most technology have the greatest moral obligation to use it wisely."

Mr. Gore pointed out that the number of peer-reviewed articles dealing with 'climate change' published in scientific journals during the previous 10 years: 928. Percentage of articles in doubt as the cause of global warming: 0%. Articles in the popular press about global warming during previous 14 years: 636. Percentage of articles in doubt as to the cause of global warming: 53%. This conclusion is that the scientific community does not have doubt as to the cause!

Rabbi Gabriel Cousens, MD, an internationally known raw food medical doctor gives a good statement about how diet relates to the environment in his book, Conscious Eating. "A conscious eating approach to a healthy diet includes going beyond our personal biochemistry to understanding diet as a way of consciously relating to the world. I call this the harmony of wholeness. It is understanding diet from the perspective of its impact on the topsoil, water supplies, air, animal population, human population, and its effect on peace in the world....The general diet that best fits with the harmony of conscious eating is vegetarian."

A Pastoral Letter on the Environment (1998) from Cardinal Law and eighteen other Bishops of New England is entitled, "And God Saw That It Was Good." After giving the Biblical basis and the Church teaching for taking care of the environment they quote another religious leader:

"Many others from Christian religious tradition have contributed to the needed public dialogue. One outstanding example of this is His All Holiness, Bartholomew I. The Ecumenical Patriarch has declared boldly, 'To commit a crime against the natural world is a sin. For humans to cause species to become extinct and to destroy the biological diversity of God's creation; for humans to degrade the integrity of the earth by causing changes in its climate, by stripping the earth of its natural forests, or destroying its wetlands; for humans to contaminate the earth's waters, its land, its air and its life with poisonous substances - these are sins.'"

We as the people of God need to accept our responsibility for our bodies and for our environment. This is a biblical mandate and also common sense. As has been noted the vegetarian diet is the best diet for both the human body and for the environment.

C. Biblical and Early Church Evidence for Jesus and Mary as a Kosher Vegetarian
(Bible is Bib question)

46. Question # Bib.46.   Is a plant-based diet seeking the Culture of Life?

The Christian is striving to move away from the world, the flesh and the devil; and towards the Kingdom of Heaven, which is among us. The penitent is involved in the Culture of Life vs. the culture of death. Pope John Paul II brought this terminology to the forefront, especially in his encyclical: *Gospel of Life*.

> "For us too, Moses' invitation rings out loud and clear: 'See, I have set before you this day life and prosperity, death and disaster' (Deut 30:15 JB) . . . 'This invitation is very appropriate for us who are called day by day to the "daily duty" of choosing between the "culture of life" and the "culture of death".'" "The Gospel of Life is at the heart of Jesus' message." "Jesus says: 'I came that they may have life, and have it abundantly' (Jn 10:10)."
> Blessed Pope John Paul II - March 25, 1995,
> The Encyclical: *Gospel of Life*, versus 28, 1.

The pilgrimage in the Culture of Life needs to recognize the importance of the penitential diet and fasting, which have been around for over 3,700 years in biblical times to the present; they are both purification methods. In the Bible the penitential diet is basically the kosher diet, it is considered a pure diet.

The biblical tradition of the Jewish people had a great emphasis on "health and healing" because the human body

72

was considered sacred. A major theme in the Hebrew Scriptures (Old Testament, 3700 - 2000 B.C.) that was central to their Jewish faith was purification or purity, expressed in another way, the clean or the unclean. This terminology was used over a 100 times in the Hebrew Scriptures. This they applied to all areas of their life because they found it keeps them healthy and able to be healed of illnesses and diseases.

The historical tradition of the Church follows this penitential tradition (or purification tradition) in the Church. In the east, the Greek Fathers tended to focus on a return to Adam's state in paradise: a recovery of the image and likeness of God (*imago Dei*) that had been lost in the fall. Gregory of Nyssa linked reform more closely to the life on earth, that is, a reformed corporeal state in the attempt to return to the original beatitude found in the Garden of Eden. An important element of renewal from the eastern fathers is the Holy Spirit's action within the heart of a human being. Basil the Great (ca. 330-79) and Cyril of Alexandria (ca. 376-444) stressed this aspect of personal reform. This emphasis is found in the first Christian community in the *Acts of the Apostles*. The Holy Spirit helps the humans in their journey to God; the Holy Spirit helps to make this trip to perfection more perfect and helps to ensure the recapturing of the *imago Dei* (image of God). The Holy Spirit role in personal reform is repeated throughout the Middle Ages and reasserted at Vatican II.

The Latin, or western, fathers also focused on a return to Adam's previous condition, but they saw something more at work. Tertullian (ca. 160-220) was the first Church Father to express the belief that the Christian receives a fuller measure of grace than Adam received because Adam lived before Christ. Jesus' resurrection brings humanity to a state beyond Adam's; Adam could never have reached this better state without Christ's redemptive death and resurrection.

The traditional stages of spiritual life are described as the Purgative way (or Purification Way) is the first stage; the second stage is the Illuminative way; and the third is the Unitive way. In theological terms these have been called: Puratrix, Illuminatrix and Perfectrix, this triad can be found as far back as St. Bonaventure. St. Bonaventure expressly calls and discusses Our Lady under the title "Purgatrix, Illuminatrix and Perfectrix" in his first sermon for the feast of the Purification (in vol. IX of the critical edition).

47. Question # Bib.47. Is a Kosher (means - pure) a Vegetarian Diet?

Biblical Kosher had three levels: 1. strict vegetarian, 2. lacto-ovo-vegetarian and 3. Kosher meat-based diets (avoiding non-kosher meats like pork, lions, bears, and others). These divisions can still be found today in the Jewish tradition in some Jewish restaurants.

Rabbi Noach Valley points out that: "In the Torah it is written, 'You shall be holy because I, Adonai your God, am holy' (Leviticus 10:2). Every one of us Jews is commanded to be holy. Holiness, in Judaism, is in the nature of an 'imitation of God.' For example, holiness and not health or hygiene is the reason for the laws of kashrut."[1]

Richard Schwartz, Ph.D. is one of the leading writers of a vegetarian Judaism. (book: *Judaism and Vegetarianism*) points out: "There is no contradiction between Judaism (and its dietary laws) and vegetarianism. In fact, Jewish vegetarians argue that vegetarianism is the diet most consistent with the highest Jewish values."[2]

The early Jewish Scriptures and lifestyle emphasized kindness to animals: "And you shall walk in His ways." Deut 28.9 "Thou shall not kill." Ex 20.13 "His (Yahweh's) compassion is over all His creatures." Ps 145.9

The words "clean" or "unclean" and "purification" or "to be purified" occur over five hundred times in the Bible, it was a major concept and concern to Biblical writers. There is a close relationship between the terms, "uncleanness" and "sin." And it was usually the priests job to "separate the sacred from the profane, the unclean from the clean."[3] The term has numerous forms such as cleanness;[4] to cleanse; to cleanse oneself; purifying; cleansing; clean; in the purifying rituals 'to sin' is normally translated as 'to cleanse'[5], and to cleanse oneself; morally clean.[6]   (cleanness (Lev 15:13; 22:4); to cleanse (Lev 16:30; Num 8:6); to cleanse oneself (Num 8:7; Josh 22:17); purifying (Lev 12:4); cleansing (Lev 13:7: Num 6:9); clean (Gen 7:2; Lev 11:47)

The unclean is prohibited or repulsive to God,[7] or it belongs to the realm of the demonic which is opposed to God, and uncleanness is described as an abomination to Yahweh. Since Yahweh was a moral God he demanded ethical purity "clean hands and a pure heart" (Ps 24:4). There is a close connection between holiness and cleanliness, but they are not the same. The Day of Atonement (a day of fasting) was specifically for the purification of the person that may be in sin or unclean. It is a day in which they were to afflict their souls (Lev 23:27, 32) by fasting (cf. Ezra 8:21) and repenting of one's sins (Ezek 18:30-31).

"The laws of kashrut can lead to a reverence for life. Yet since the blood is the life of the body, Jews are forbidden to eat blood. 'For the life of the flesh is in the blood.' (Lev 17:11) By this verse alone some Jews may have been a vegetarian even during Passover. While most Jewish scholars assume that all Jews ate meat during the time that the Temple stood, it is significant that some (Tosafot, Yoma 3a, and Rabbeinu, Sukkah 42b) assert that even during the Temple period it was not an absolute requirement to eat meat."[8]

The prohibition against eating blood was extremely important and even foreigners were not exempt (Lev 12:10-

12). There is always a tiny amount of blood even if the animals were drained of the blood. So the best way to stay pure and 'clean' was to avoid any animal meat that has blood in it, which basically means all land animal meats and meat products. The Torah Laws are to help us get back to a plant-based lifestyle that was found with Adam and Eve. The New Testament brings forth the new Adam and Eve, Jesus and his Blessed Mother Mary.

The teaching of the clean and the unclean was known in New Testament times as is indicated when Jesus used the parable of the dragnet to distinguish between the good fish and the bad fish as found in the Torah teaching on Kosher. "Once again, the kingdom of heaven is like a net that was let down into the lake and caught all kinds of fish. When it was full, the fishermen pulled it up on the shore. Then they sat down and collected the good fish in baskets, but threw the bad away." Mt 13:47, 48

Purification is a key biblical and New Testament concept.
- Christianity began with the Aramaic phrase: "Purify thyself and believe the Good News." Mk 1:15
- "He has clean hands and a pure heart." Psalms 24:4
- "I have made my heart clean. I am pure." Prov 20:9
- "Blessed are the pure in heart," Matt 5:8
- "Purify your hearts." James 4:8
- "Seeing ye have purified your souls." 1 Peter 1:22
- "thou will show thyself pure." 2 Samuel 22:27; Psalm 18;26
- "He shall purify himself." Num 19:12
- "many shall be purified and made white." Dan 12:10
- "Every word of God is pure." Prov. 30:5
- "Purifying himself." Acts 21:26;
- "Sanctified to the purifying of the flesh." Heb 9:13
- "Keep thyself pure …" 1 Tim 5:22
- "Unto the pure all things are pure;" Titus 1:15
- "The wisdom that is from above is first pure." Ja 3:17

As the famous 5th century monk Dionysius the Areopagite says, "Purified souls, being raised up to the heights of contemplation, participate in the Divine, 'Thus do we learn that it is the Cause and Origin and Being and Life of all creation. (Gen 1) It is a Principle of Illumination to them that are being enlightened; a Principle of Perfection to them that are being perfected; a principle of Deity to them that are being deified; and of Simplicity to them that are being brought into simplicity.'[a]"[9]

48. Question # Bib.48   Is there a study on a Toxicology Study on the Torah and Meat?

A fascinating study by a researcher looking at Leviticus XI and Deuteronomy XIV, gives some scientific support for God's wisdom. "Much of the wisdom in the Divine Design for meats was confirmed by a 1953 study in which Dr. David Macht of Johns Hopkins University reported the toxic effects of animal flesh on a controlled growth culture."[10] "His results show that the lower the growth percentage of the culture, the more toxic the flesh. Note that the flesh of animals and fish given to us by God for food are all nontoxic, but all forbidden animals lie in the toxic range."[11]

"His results show that the lower the growth percentage of the culture, the more toxic the flesh. Note that the flesh of animals and fish given to us by God for food are all nontoxic, but all forbidden animals lie in the toxic range." Animals without percentage rankings in the chart were not studied, but are included here to provide a more comprehensive list of clean and unclean meats. "Don't get confused! Any number above 75 percent is nontoxic,

---

[a] Illumination: as in Purgation, Illumination and Union. Perfection: technical usage as in 1 Cor. 2:6; Phil. 3:15. Deity: as St. Bernard bluntly says: "To experience this state is to be deified."   Simplicity: soul turns from complex world to having one desire - for God, in a simple and unified state, Mat 6:22.

or clean."[12]

Quadrupeds (Four Footed)
Clean (Cloven-hoofed and cud chewing) - calf (82%); deer (98%); goat (90%); ox (91%); sheep (94%).

Unclean - black bear (59%); camel (41%); cat (62%); guinea pig (46%); dog (62%); fox (58%); grizzly bear (55%); ground hog (53%); hamster (46%); horse (39%); opossum (53%); rabbit (49%); rat (55%); rhinoceros (60%); squirrel (43%); swine (54%).

Birds
Clean - goose (85%); chicken (83%); coot (88%); duck (98%); pigeon (93%); quail (89%); swan (87%); turkey (85%).

Unclean - bat; cormorant; crow (46%); eagle; falcon; hawk; heron; ibis; kite; nighthawk; osprey; ostrich; owl (62%); pelican; raven red-tail hawk (36%); sparrow hawk (63%); sea gull; stork, vulture.

Fish
Clean (with scales and fins) - black bass (80%); black drum (105%); bluefish (80%); carp (90%); channel bass (80%); chub (91%); cod (98%); croaker (90%); flounder (83%); flying fish (87%); goldfish (88%); haddock (80%); hake (98%); halibut (82%); herring (100%); kingfish (83%); mullet (87%); pike (98%); pompano (110%); porgy (80%); rainbow trout (81%); rock bass (100%); salmon (81%); smelt (90%); sea bass (103%); shad (100%); Spanish mackerel (98%); spot (80%); sturgeon (87%); tuna (88%); white perch (81%); carolina whiting (84%); yellow perch 87%).

Unclean (without scales and fins) - catfish (48%); clams; crabs; eel (40%); lobster; octopus; oysters; porcupine fish (60%); puffer (51%); sand skate (59%); scallops; shark (62%); shrimp; squid; stingray (46%); toad fish (49%).

Basic science would indicate that animals who eat other animals would have a higher toxic percentage then animals who ate leaves and grass. Animals store toxins and poisons in their fat cells and the more animals, other animals eat, the higher the toxin rate in their cells. The Biblical Jews on the subject of kosher were in line with the modern biochemistry and toxicology!

In the Old Testament, the dietary principles of a pure diet (Kosher) are basically that they are allowed to eat the "clean" vegetarian animals (sheep, goat, ox, etc.) and not allowed to eat the 'unclean' meat eating animals (lions, bears, wolves, etc.) or the scavenger animals (pigs, wild boars, sharks, clams, shrimp, etc.). God was showing his people which meats were safe and which meats were unsafe, from the biblical teachings. The unclean are connected to sin and evil that can come upon the people as with Numbers 11. Another obvious text: "Do not make yourself detestable with all these crawling beasts; do not defile yourself with them, do not be defiled by them; 'For it is I, Yahweh, who am your God.' You have been sanctified and have become holy because I am holy; do not defile yourself with all these beasts that crawl on the ground." Lev 11:43, 44

49. Question # Bib.49 What about Jesus and Mary; were they beautiful and clean inwardly, physiologically purified?

Was the Virgin Mary's arteries corroded; her nerves in knots; her liver and kidneys clogged up; the walls of her colon all coated with grime; her toxicity level high; her blood contaminated and other physiological problems?

Both Jesus Christ and the Blessed Virgin Mary were physiologically clean, purified and beautiful inside her body. Beautiful skin and complexion is often one of the many fruits of being clean or purified inside. His and her skin and complexion would have been clean and beautiful outside too! In her many apparitions she radiated beauty. "It is said that Pope Leo XIII, the great faster, had a very clear, almost transparent complexion."[13]

50. Question # Bib.50   What are the Kings Delicacies?

A good example of the effects of 'the kings delicacies' foods are found in the mummies of Egypt. Dr. Rex Russell, M.D. points out: "We have a clear idea of the Egyptian diseases from radiographs and autopsies performed on mummies by paleopathologist Marc A. Ruffer and others.[14] These studies show that many Egyptians had the same diseases that still cause illness today. The most common affliction of the Egyptians appears to be vascular diseases that resulted in severely calcified arteries. Other common maladies included arthritis, tooth decay, infections, cancer, emphysema, tuberculosis, parasites, pneumonia and obesity. Childbirth deaths and infections afterbirth were also fairly common. Mummified Pharaohs often show the most advanced degenerative diseases. Historically, Pharaohs and other royalty (see 1 Kg 4:22ff; Amos 6:4) were the only ones whose diets included large quantities of meat and other delicacies."[15]

'"When you sit down to dine with a ruler, keep in mind who is before you; put a knife to your throat if you have a ravenous appetite. Do not desire his delicacies; they are deceitful food." Prov 23.1-3 'Let not my heart be drawn to what is evil, to take part in wicked deeds with men who are evildoers; let me not eat of their delicacies." Ps 141:4

"Food, of course cannot bring us in touch with God: we lose nothing if we refuse to eat, we gain nothing if we eat. Take care, however, lest in exercising your right you become an occasion of sin to the weak." "Therefore, if food causes my brother [or sister] to sin I will never eat meat again, so that I may not be an occasion of sin to him [her]." 1 Cor. 8:8, 9, 13

51. Question # Bib.51   What were the biblical three Altars of the Lord?

In the Old Testament the Jewish people lived a simple lifestyle and they had three main altars that bring life, that were sacred to them.

- The first is the sacred altar of sacrifice; this was the forerunner of the Eucharistic table.
- The second the sacred altar was the altar of the marriage bed which brings forth new life in children.
- The third sacred altar was the kitchen table, since it brings forth life through health and avoiding sickness. At the kitchen table they only served kosher foods, kosher means 'pure' and pure foods imply that it is life-giving. All Jews at that time were kosher, it was part of who they were.

Rev. Lawrence E. Frizzell[16] in his *Marian Studies* (1995) article, "Mary and the Biblical Heritage" is helping us at "Refreshing our memory concerning the patterns of piety in the Jewish home and larger community will help us to model our lives on the examples of Jesus and his Mother."[17] Concerning the Temple and the Commandments there is a triad of piety found in the biblical text concerning their lifestyle (sacred altar of sacrifice; kosher kitchen table/altar; marriage bed altar). Lawrence Frizzell cites the work by Jacob Neusner, *The Idea of Purity in Judaism*,[18] and gives the pattern of piety that was three-fold paradigm: the Temple-worship purification and its daily rhythms of prayer at home and in the synagogue; the food laws to grow in purity since the body is sacred; and the commandments concerning sex in marriage as pure.

Fr. Frizzell adds, "Would the people of Nazareth grasp that the preparation of food (with its emphasis on the responsibility of farmer and housewife) enabled those partaking of a meal to experience God's presence? If they did not express the experience, Luke certainly understood the spiritual significance of a meal (e.g., Lk 14:1-24; 22:1-20; 24:13-25). The prophets Hosea (Ch 1-3), Jeremiah (2:1; 3:10) and Ezekiel (16:1-63) stressed that marriage is a paradigm in the human order that provides a basis for their teaching about the covenant between God and his people."[19]

52. Question # Bib.52   Were Jesus and Mary the New Adam and Eve?

Mary belongs to an Order of Eden[20] (*Marian Studies*) which is about the line of succession and linage from Adam and Eve to Mary's Jewish Essene parents and her uniqueness as the New Eve, and as the Daughter of Zion (Zephaniah 3.14-17) because she qualifies as a personification of the elect people, the "kosher woman." It is the Virgin Mary's privilege, analogically, to belong to an Order of Eden! The linage of Eve goes to Mary as Our Lady of Eden. The first prophecy (Gen 3:15) spoke of the woman (Mary) who with her Seed would repair the order of the fall in Eden. Thus St. Jerome (300 AD) quotes: "Death through Eve; life through Mary," which is a theme picked up by St. Augustine and other Church Fathers. Jesus and Mary have become the new Adam and Eve.

The New Testament texts that connect Jesus and Adam include: Rom 5:14-19 also the verse "Just as in Adam all die, so in Christ all will come to life again." 1 Co 15:21, 22 "Scripture has it that Adam, the first man, became a living soul; the last Adam became a life-giving spirit. … so shall we bear the likeness of the man from heaven." 1 Cor 15:45-49 The parallel of Adam to Jesus is presented nine times in the New Testament and led to the association of Eve to Mary. The post-apostolic Fathers St. Justin (155) and St. Irenaeus, (circa 177) both write on the Eve-Mary parallel. Other Church Fathers also compare Mary with Eve.[21] Irenaeus sees both Christ and Mary as untying the very knot that Adam and Eve had bound together through their disobedience, which started with food.[22]

We can approximate their plant-based diet, especially since many studies have shown the health and healing benefits of a plant-based diet. Furthermore since the new-Adam and new-Eve, Jesus and Mary, ate a plant-based diet and fasted, from the present research available,[23] it encourages us to look into this possibility. Adam and Eve are the ideal examples of a raw vegan diet. Jesus and Mary were the new Adam and Eve.

Professor Roberta Kalechofsky Ph.D.,[24] points out that: "The first law of kashruth is, in fact, the commandment to be vegetarian: 'God said, "See, I give you all the seed-bearing plants that are upon the whole earth, and all the trees with seed-bearing fruit; this shall be your food.'" Gen 1:29

53. Question # Bib.53 Was Jesus the Vegetarian Messiah?

The most famous prophecy of the Messiah is Isaiah 7:14, 15. "Therefore the Lord himself will give you this sign: the virgin shall be with child, and bear a son, and shall name him Immanuel. He shall be living on curds and whey by the time he learns to reject the bad and choose the good."

"He shall be living on curds and whey" is a prophecy of the Messiah, a prophecy indicating that he Jewish Messiah was to be brought up as a vegetarian. Curds and whey are a vegetarian protein similar to yogurt or kefier. Thus the Immanuel shall be brought up as a vegetarian.

The famous Rabbi Abraham Isaac Kook (1865-1935) the first Chief Rabbi of pre-state Israel was a great scholar and advocate of vegetarianism. He was one of the major influences of modern Jewish vegetarianism. According to Rabbi Kook, the people in the time of Noah had sunk to an extremely low level of spirituality and thus they were given the elevated image of themselves as compared to animals.

The blood laws are part of the Torah that the Messiah must follow. As the Messiah, he would have had to follow every dot and iota of the law, including vegetarian kosher. Jesus was vegetarian and upheld it in order to fulfill the teachings of the Torah, God's Word. In Mosaic Law, blood must be strictly separated from food. (Lev 3:17; 7:26-27; 17:3-7; 10B14; 19:26; Deut 12:15-16, 20-28; 15:19-23; 1 Sam 14:32-35; Ex 33:25)

The Messiah must follow the Laws and not turn to the right or to the left of these commandments. (Deut. 17:20) This would include the laws that concern blood, the Messiah must not partake of the blood of any animal during his life. After the resurrection Jesus had a resurrected body and did partake of a piece of fish for the sake of the disciples.

54. Question # Bib.54 Was Jesus a Physician?

Jesus may have been brought up as a carpenter, but the evidence suggests that he later became versed in the healing arts and became a well-known physician. Jesus knew the Essenes and the Therapeutae Jewish communities, who are strong in the healing arts. Origen, an early Church Father asserts that Jesus was not a carpenter as he grew up, '. . . that in none of the Gospels current in the Churches is Jesus Himself ever described as being a carpenter.' The oldest translation of Mark 6 states, "Jesus son of Joseph the carpenter," later translations write, Jesus the carpenter, son of Joseph. Twice Jesus referred to himself as a physician: Lk 4:23, Mk 2:15-17 which are confirmed in parallel text Mk 2.17 and Lk 5:32. Jesus spent about a third or more of his time healing people in the Gospels. Finally, some of the early Church Fathers called Jesus the Divine physician.

Dealing with diet, fasting and herbs would have been the main part of Jesus work as a physician in biblical times. He was well aware of the kosher laws and the benefits of a plant-based lifestyle and its healing properties and would have promoted that. Mary watching her son would have been aware of this too. Both of them lived in a Nazarene community that was vegetarian and promoted these values.

55. Question # Bib.55   Was Jesus an Essene?

A New Testament use of the Essenes is found as the Scribes, a religious party. "In Gospel material formulated relatively late, the scribes are independently named alongside the Pharisees (Mark 7:1, 5; Matt. 5:20; 12:38; 15:1; 23:2; Luke 5:21; 6:7; 11:53; 15:2; John 8:3) and are therefore reckoned as a group to be distinguished from the latter. On the other hand, there were occasionally "Scribes who belonged to the Pharisee party" (Mark 2:16; cf. John 3:1-12; 7:50-52; 19:39) and perhaps also scribes who were members of none of the great religious parties. In any case, the group designation 'scribes' strongly suggest the thought of the Essenes as the elite group in Judaism at that time, even after the destruction of the Temple. The oldest of our Gospels independently names, alongside the Pharisees, also the Herodians (Mark 3:6; 12:13; cf. 8:15; Matt. 22:16)."[25]

The name that Jesus was commonly known was "Jesus the Nazorean"[b] and also "Jesus the Nazarene"[c]. The term Nazarene describes a person who came from the town of Nazareth, which Jesus did.[d] The Nazarites were a branch of the Essenes and about 16 times Jesus is referred to as in this manner of a Nazarite or a Nazorean, directly relating him to the Essenes, put simply Jesus was an Essene. The Virgin Mary's parent were Essenes according to the visionary Blessed Catherine Emmerick. Mary and Jesus were brought up in their tradition and were vegetarians.

---

[b] (Mt 2:23; 26:71: Lk 18:37; Jn 18:5, 7; 19:19; Ac 2:22; 3:6; 4:10; 6:14; 22:8; 26:9; cf. 9:5)

[c] (Mk 1:24; 10:47; 14:67; 16;6; Lk 4:34; 24:19)

[d] (Mt 21:11; Jn 1:45-46; Ac 10:38; cf. Mk 1:9; Lk 4:16)

56. Question # Bib.56 What did Josephus and Philo write about the Essenes?

Josephus and Philo were scholars and historians whose writings were around New Testament times. The Nazoreans (Ac 24:5; cf. Ac 24:14, 28:22); the Sadducees (Ac 5:17), the Pharisees (Ac 15:5, 26:5) and the Essenes (Josephus: *The Life* 2 sec.10) are all characterized as 'Sects' of Judaism. The writers who mentioned the Essenes are: Philo, Pliny, Dio Chrysostom, Josephus, Hippolytus and Epiphanius. Josephus claims to have spent time with the Essenes at age 16 (ca. 53-54 CE). Josephus writes about three "Jewish philosophical schools" in this period: the Sadducees, the Pharisee's and the Essenes.[26]

Josephus says of the Essenes, "they were stricter than all Jews in not undertaking work on the seventh day" and they held Moses in greatest reverence.[27] They were very interested in the study of the "holy books" and other ancient writings in order to "search out medicinal roots and the properties of stones" to heal diseases.[28] The Essenes held angels in importance and they also gave prophecy in the community. And the Essenes believed in bodily resurrection,[29] and in everlasting life,[30] and in Messianic Apocalypse.[31] Philo says they ate "bread and vegetables".

Obviously one of the four footed animal that is unclean is the swine or pig. Yes, ham and bacon and other meat products from pigs are unclean and the Jews back then took this very seriously as a sin and some still do today.

"The Hebrew word for 'meat' (basar) was explained by the Talmudists with the following acronym: bet: shame, sin: corruption, resh: worms. The more flesh, the more worms." [32] This connects meat directly with sin.

Philo and Josephus are two Jewish historians who lived and wrote around the time of Christ. Kosher food was of great importance for the Essenes and most of the early sects of Judaism. It was so important that they would die for it. "Philo reports that Jewish women were offered 'swine's flesh' and tortured if they refused to eat it during anti-Jewish riots in Alexandria ca. 38 C.E."[33]

"According to Josephus, the Romans tortured the Essenes during the first Jewish revolt (66-74 C.E.) for refusing to renounce the dietary rules: 'They were racked and twisted, burnt and broken, and made to pass through every instrument of torture in order to induce them to blaspheme their lawgiver and to eat some forbidden thing. Yet, they refused to yield to either demand, nor even once did they cringe to their persecutors or shed a tear. Smiling in their agonies, mildly deriding their tormentors, they cheerfully resigned their souls, confident that they would receive them back again."[34]

Josephus refers to a certain company of Jewish priests who "being truly pious towards God supported themselves on figs and nuts," a reference to a vegetarian diet that was an Essene custom.[35] Jesus was a Nazarite (from Joseph) and Mary was an Essene from her mother Joachim and Anne, (confirmed by mystic Anne Catherine Emmerick's visions in her books) they were part of the larger Essene community.

Josephus refers to a certain company of priests who "being truly pious towards God supported themselves on figs and nuts", a reference to a vegetarian diet that was an Essene custom.[36] "Fasting was a regular Jewish custom, observed by the reforming sects also (cf. Mark 2:18). The duty of observing the 'day of fast' is mentioned in CD 6:19, along with 'distinguishing between clean and unclean, making known between the holy and the profane, observing the Sabbath according to its interpretation and the feasts....'"[37]

The Qumran disciplines were an attempt at a radical transformation of the human condition to a healthier and holier state of life. Part of this effort to become "another man" (1 Sam 10:6) is the experience of ecstasy and other uplifted states of consciousness. Ecstatic behavior was often associated with prophecy. (1 Sam 10:5-13) Prophecy was part of the Essenes as noted by Josephus[38] and the Therapetae were noted by Philo for their strong ecstatic element. The prophets were credited with miracles and healing diseases (1 Kgs 17:10-24; 2 Kgs 4:8-37; Isa 38:1-8; Num 21:6-9). Jesus was also thought to be a prophet because of his healing miracles as in Mark 1:27; 6:2-4, 14-15, etc. The Essenes were also known for their healing arts.

"According to Philo and other authors of that time the Essenes were vegetarians (also confirmed by modern historians such as Robert Eisenman, PhD) and took no drink other than rainwater or the juice of fruits. It is said that their diet was fruits, vegetables, nuts, seeds, and grains."[39]

57. Question # Bib.57   Is Christianity Related to or a Continuation of the Essenes?

One scholar of the Dead Sea Scrolls, Upton Ewing, in his book, *The Prophet of the Dead Sea Scrolls,* gives a rather convincing set of reasons on this topic. "Accordingly, so-called 'Palestinian Christianity' can be better understood historically as a continuation of, rather than an outgrowth of so-called 'Essenism.' The seven points which further illustrate this to be true are as set forth in the following premises:"[40]

(1) "That these devoutly religious people were the only ones in their part of the world whose common custom was evidenced by the wearing of a single white garment.

(2) That they were the only sect in their part of the world who practiced an economy whereby everything was held in common.

(3) That they were the only people in their part of the world whose religious leaders, or priesthood, practiced celibacy.

(4) That they were the only sect in their part of the world who opposed the custom of slavery.

(5) That they were the only religious sect, not alone in their own country but in the entire Roman world, who opposed the custom of animal sacrifice.

(6) That they were the only people in Palestine or of the greater Roman world who opposed the slaughter of animals for food.

(7) That they were the only people of Palestine and the outside Roman world whose way of life was opposed to war and the soldier' calling."[41]

All of these groups lived in the same general area of Galilee and the Dead Sea, in a way they were neighboring towns and villages. They were all orthodox Jews with basically the same Jewish beliefs and practices. As neighbors and friends they all interacted and may have even worked and worshiped together at times. There is no indication in the literature that these groups (Essenes, Nazarenes, Therapeutae) were at odds with one another but there is indication that these groups were at odds with the Pharisees and Sadducees in Jerusalem. These groups were really one large group of closely associated sects such that they were one sect, different branches on the same tree. And the trunk of that tree could be called the Essenes. This is the community that Jesus and Mary grew up in.

Rabbi Gabriel Cousens, MD a modern day Jewish Essene, gives some good insight.[42] ; "The Essene Archetype is a very intriguing, inspiring ideal. The ancient Essenes were historically recognized as the mystical Jewish prophets of the desert. They considered themselves, in their terms, 'the holy ones of God'. It is no accident that the term *Essene* comes from the Northern Aramaic word *chasya*, which means *saint* in Greek, which was the way they were perceived by the general population. From the time of Hannokh they were also known as *B'nei Aliyah*, the children of ascension. Many of the early Jewish followers of Jesus were also Essene; it is also strongly suggested historically that Mary's parents (Joachim and Anna), Jesus' parents (Mary and Joseph), his brother James, and John the Baptist were also Essene. In 2007, at an Easter talk,[43] Pope Benedict XVI acknowledged that the home were Jesus had his last meal was an Essene home, and his second volume of *Jesus of Nazareth* (2011) mentions the Essenes in general and in specific in the context of Jesus' 'Last Supper.'[44] This suggests that Jesus was clearly associated with the Essenes. If he was not formally trained as an Essene as some historians suggest, he was at least close to them in some spiritual and lifestyle alignment. The Essene existence is first mentioned about 500 B.C., after the fall of the First Temple in 586 B.C., in Pythagora's biography, where he studied with them on Mt. Carmel and came down enlightened and as a teacher of live foods [raw vegans]. These were called the Galilean Essenes of the north, where Jesus came from. The Galilean Essenes were also given the name Nazarenes, as was Jesus."[45]

"The Essenes lived in various communities all over the Middle East. They totaled in number between 4,000 to 10,000 people. This included the Qumran Essene community, which began in 186 B.C. near the Dead Sea. There were also Essenes at the Sea of Galilee, Mt. Carmel, in Egypt at Lake Mareotis, as well as in the areas that are now known as Lebanon and Damascus. These Essene groups, which resided all over the region, had slightly different styles according to the local culture, but shared the basics of Essene life and spirituality. They believed in creating a lifestyle that would support the human transformation into a whole and healthy life. They were noted by the historian Philo, for their focus on living ecstatically. They lived strictly and honorably by these ethics. Historical evidence indicates that the vast majority of the Essenes adhered to a plant-source-only and/ or live-foods diet."[46]

Cardinal Ratzinger and the Pontifical Biblical Commission (2001) released a document: *The Jewish People and Their Sacred Scriptures in the Christian Bible*, it speaks

several times of the Essenes. They connect the Essene community with the new covenant school of thought: "the Qumran group formed the community of the new covenant."[47] The Commission makes the connection between the Essenes and the Christian message; and point out that the theology of Jesus is closer to the Essenes. "His belief in angels and the resurrection of the body, as well as the eschatological expectation attributed to him in the Gospels, is much closer to the theology of the Essenes and the Pharisees."[48] Whereas Cardinal Joseph Ratzinger stopped short of stating that Jesus was an Essene, he did state later as Pope Benedict in his book, *Jesus of Nazareth*,[49] "The earnest religiosity of the Qumran writings is moving; it appears that not only John the Baptist, but possibly Jesus and his family as well, were close to the Qumran community. At any rate, there are numerous points of contact with the Christian message in the Qumran writings. It is a reasonable hypothesis that John the Baptist lived for some time in this community and received part of his religious formation
from it."[50]

58. Question # Bib.58 Was the Essene Jerusalem Community Kosher and Vegetarian?

There is only one mention of the Virgin Mary in the Acts of the Apostles, after the ascension they returned to Jerusalem. "Together they devoted themselves to constant prayer. There were some women in their company, and Mary the mother of Jesus, and his brethren." Acts 1:14 Then at Pentecost it is written, "All were filled with the Holy Spirit" and "They devoted themselves to the apostle's instruction and the communal life, to the breaking of bread and the prayers. A reverent fear overtook them all, for many wonders and signs were performed by the
Apostles." Ac 2:4, 42, 43.

Mary the mother of Jesus was involved in the beginning of the Jerusalem Community. This community was centered in Jerusalem but was scattered in towns and villages around Jerusalem and throughout Galilee; whether she lived in Jerusalem or more likely in one of the neighboring towns or back in her home town of Nazareth, she would have been part of the Jerusalem community, their beliefs and practices. The Kosher orientation of the Jerusalem community was one of their main Jewish practices. Mary the Mother of Jesus would have been kosher all this time. Some mystics (i.e. either Blessed Anne Catherine Emmerick, Venerable Mary of Agreda; St. Bridget of Sweden; or St. Elizabeth of Schoenau.[51] on the following quote) describe the Virgin Mary as a vegetarian. "She ate very sparingly and took no meat, though she prepared it for Joseph. She usually ate cooked vegetables and bread, fruit and fish."[52]

In Pope Benedict XVI (Pope in 2005) book *Jesus of Nazareth,*[53] he writes on the possible community connections of the family of Jesus: "An accidental discovery after the Second World War led to excavation at Qumran, which brought to light texts that some scholars have associated with yet another movement known until then only from literary references: the so-called Essenes. This group had turned its back on the Herodian temple and its worship to withdraw to the Judean desert. There it created monastic-style communities, but also a religiously motivated common life for families. It also established a productive literary center and instituted distinctive rituals, which included liturgical ablutions and common prayers. The earnest religiosity of the Qumran writings is moving. It appears that not only John the Baptist, but possibly Jesus and his family as well, were close to the Qumran community. At any rate, there are numerous points of contact with the Christian message in the Qumran writings. It is a reasonable hypothesis that John the Baptist lived for some time in this community and received part of his religious formation from it."[54]

In Acts 6:7 we read: "The word of God continued to spread, while the same time the number of the disciples in Jerusalem enormously increased. There were many priests among those who embraced the faith." Who were these many priests who embraced the faith? Surely they were not the Pharisees and Sadducees! This means that these priests who embraced the faith were from the Essene group: the Essenes, the Therapeutae and the Nazarites and others all under the umbrella of the Essenes.

The Essenes seemed to have disappeared a century or so after Jesus death and at the same time the followers of 'the Way' Christianity grew enormously during this same time period. Jesus spent only a week or two in Jerusalem and nearly all of his time in the greater Galilee area where the Essenes were located, around 4,000 of them yet another estimate has been around 10,000, it depends on how much the sects are included in the count. Perhaps many of these converts to Christianity came from the Essenes, Therapeutae and the Nazarenes, who were all looking for the coming of the Messiah. Perhaps this is why the Essenes disappeared a century after Jesus death because most if not all of them became the first Christians.

In the Jewish tradition at the time of Jesus and Mary, there could be said to be three types of Jews regarding diet: 1) those who disregarded the Old Testament teachings on diet and ate whatever they liked; 2) those who were kosher and ate kosher meat and dairy according to the Old Testament laws and 3) those who were vegetarian kosher and either were partially vegetarian or strict vegetarian; this may have included lacto-ovo vegetarians who had milk (unpasteurized thus still a healthy alkaline state) and fresh eggs, it also had vegans, and probably 80/20 raw vegans. Over a hundred years later because of the persecution of the Jews, the term Kosher was rejected by many early Christians.

Thus it would have been extremely easy for Jesus and Mary to have been Kosher and even vegetarian among these groups of people, since it was the lifestyle of most of these Essene Jews and a widely accepted dietary practice in this area. This area was a Garden of Eden with all the groves and gardens back in biblical times, the heat wave and climate changes didn't happen for about 500 years turning Israel into a desert type of country. They had access to much produce, fruit trees, vines, vegetables, grains, nuts, seeds and herbs.

According to the ancient historian Josephus, the Pharisees and the Sadducees were two of the three groups of priests, the third was the Essenes. The Essenes were strict kosher, mostly vegetarian kosher after the Biblical Laws. The Essenes had a lot of priests and apparently many of them joined the disciples, this is why when Jesus entered Jerusalem and other areas he had many followers, some priests. The Essenes refused to sacrifice animals in the Temple and once a year made an offering of fruits, breads and vegetables.

"Jewish groups, dedicated wholly to the study and observance of the Law, and living a pious, ascetic and communal life, were held up for admiration in antiquity not only by Jewish writers life Phio[55] and Josephus,[56] but even by Gentiles like the roman Pliny the Elder.[57] The Jerusalem community described in the early part of Acts bears notable resemblance to these idealized groups. As more and more of the Dead Sea scrolls become available from scholars, comparisons between some aspects of the life of the Qumran communities and the earliest church have been attempted, a number of studies tried to relate the communal meals of Acts 2:42-7 to the religious common meal of the Dead Sea community. [58"59]

59. Question # Bib.59 Did the First Jewish-Christian Communities Considered Jesus a Vegetarian?

Professor Kalechofsky, PhD writes: "With the fall of Jerusalem in 70 C.E. came the destruction of the Temple and the disappearance of priestly slaughterers. "Above all, an enormous sense of mourning must have hung over the surviving remnant. A mourner loses his appetite and his interest in the joys of living. For the expression of these feelings, a number of mourners must have been attracted to the ascetic cults of ancient Israel, which had already existed for quite some time before the destruction. The Qumran group associated with the Dead Sea Scrolls appears to have already disappeared, but there were others - Nazirites, Rechabites, Essenes, Therapeutae, and Zakokites. With the destruction of the Temple, the ascetic cults must have expressed as never before a predominant mood of the people. A central feature of some of these ascetic groups was abstinence from the eating of meat. Celibacy, fasting, and other forms of privation also marked the ascetic regimen, but vegetarianism was a prominent symbol of the ascetic life, and was now fittingly associated with mourning for the destruction of the Temple."[60] "Following the destruction of the Temple, the number of recluses who would not eat meat or drink wine increased in Israel."[61]

Some orthodox Jewish writers recognize that in order to fulfill the laws of the Torah the vegetarian lifestyle was the ideal.[62] All of these groups lived in the same general area of Galilee, Nazareth, and the Dead Sea. They all had similar beliefs and practices, they were neighbors and friends. Jesus lived with, ate with, preached too and taught many of these early communities.

In the *Encyclopedia of the Early Church*, the Church Fathers[63] wrote that certain groups abstained from particular foods including: the Encratites, Ebionites, Marcionites, Manichaeans, and Priscillianists, who seem to have considered Jesus a vegetarian.[64]

"Origen says that these Jews who have received Jesus Christ were all called by the name 'Ebionites'"[65] And St. Epipanius (ca. 350) writes that "the Ebionite Sect was in existence (35 CE)."[66] Bishop Epiphanius (A.D. 315-403) of Constantia in Cyprus, in his book *Panarion*[67] states,

'Whenever you speak to them (Ebionites) concerning flesh food, the Ebionites reply they were vegetarian because "Christ revealed it to me.'[68] This is another reference connecting the Ebionites to the early Christians.

According to the *Encyclopedia of the Dead Sea Scrolls* it writes: "In the second and third centuries, the Church Fathers Irenaeus (c. 130-200 CE), Clement of Alexandria (c. 150-215 CE) and Hippolytus (c. 170-236 CE) applied that name Encratites to a diverse array of early Christian groups adopting ascetic practices such as celibacy, abstinence from wine, and vegetarianism. Particularly important is an organized Jewish-Christian community that, according to Irenaeus,[69] was founded in the latter part of the second century in Mesopotamia by Tatian.

Tatian was a pupil of Justin Martyr (c. 100-165 CE) and author of the Diatessaron (a famous harmony of the four canonical Gospels). Justin Martyr was involved in Christianity during the beginning of the early Church and surely would have known the Apostle John. The Encratite community that Tatian founded was vegetarian which means that Justin was probably a vegetarian himself or at least approved of it.

This is significant to have this witness on vegetarianism so close to the original Christian community in Jerusalem. The connection here is important. Tatian was a disciple of Justin Martyr. Justin was probably a disciple of the Apostle John, and John took care of Mary, which implies that perhaps Justin, John and Mary were vegetarian or at least approved of it!

The Virgin Mary and Jesus lived among these people for probably 25 years, assuming they were in Egypt for only five years, where they probably would have been associated with the Jewish Essene community called the Therapeutae in Egypt, who were versed in the healing arts. Then when Jesus started his ministry, the majority of the time he spent in this greater area of Galilee, except for the short times he spent preaching in Jerusalem. Thus Jesus was preaching to and eating with many of the people in these Jewish sects: the Nazarene's, the Essenes, the Ebionites, the Therapeutae's and others who were strict kosher and even vegetarian. In addition, almost all of his disciples and followers came from these groups, which were mostly or totally vegetarian. And those after Jesus time, continued with the vegetarian tradition, such as the Titan community mentioned above.

The Church Fathers[70] had some good insights into fasting. The Christian fasts spiritually by abstaining from evil,[71] observing the commandments, confiding in God and serving him with a pure heart; fasting from food will help the poor: 'on the day of the fast, eat only bread and water and, working out the cost of the food you would have consumed, give a corresponding sum to a widow, an orphan, a needy person'.[72] The whole family will take part with joy: 'Observe these things with your children and all your household: thus you will be happy".[73]

Abstinence is a partial fast, esp. from meat and wine, which allows us to survive and hence to fast again.[74] It is ascesis, not aversion to diabolical foods.[75] Certain groups abstained from particular foods: Encratites, Ebionites, Marcionites, Manichaeans, Priscillianists, who seem to have considered Jesus a vegetarian.[76] Some claimed that St Peter "ate only bread, olives and herbs"[77].

Clement of Alexandria (b. circa AD 150), was a well educated teacher, in his *Paidagogos* a handbook of Christian etiquette in the practical needs of life to eating, drinking and table manners. Clement's aim throughout the treatise is to inculcate the virtue of temperance. Clement also appeals to medical opinion and cites Antiphanes, "a Delian physician, for the assertion that rich food is one of the causes of diseases."[78]

"The Law was wise, he stresses, to prohibit rich food, which, in addition to being unhealthy and fattening, engenders greed, is expensive, and absorbs attention and resources that are better spent elsewhere. Phio (a Jewish historian) interpreted the Jewish dietary law both literally and symbolically. Following him, Clement sees great wisdom in the Law by which the Lord announced a long time ago that 'we are to exercise control over the belly, and what is below the belly' and which still teaches us 'patience and self restraint' by 'repressing our desires'. The Law is still useful for checking lust and condemning pleasure. Clement recommends to his philosophic Christians to avoid 'such articles of food as excite lust and dissolute licentiousness in the bed chamber and luxury'."[79]

One of the primary reasons that these Jewish people in community became vegetarian and upheld it was to fulfill the teachings of the Torah, God's Word. In Mosaic Law, blood must be strictly separated from food. (Lev 3:17; 7:26-27; 17:3-7; 10B14; 19:26; Deut 12:15-16, 20-28; 15:19-23; 1 Sam 14:32-35; Ex 33:25) The prohibition against eating blood was extremely important and even foreigners were not exempt (Lev 12:10-12). The easy way, in fact the only way to truly fulfill this requirement was to be vegetarian and not eat any meat that has blood in it.

60. Question # Bib.60 Were the Nazarenes Vegetarians?

Some in the Catholic Church see the writings of Bishop Epiphanius of Salamis as Gnostic writings but others would see it as a historical document of the 4th century. Putting these disputes aside let us look at the writing itself.

When the holy family fled to Egypt they fled to the Essene community of the "theraputae" or "healers" at Lake Mareotis, in Egypt. This community is described by the historian and Jewish philosopher Philo. Jesus was primarily associated with the Esenes of Mount Carmel in Northern Israel, not the Essenes of Qumran in Southern Israel. Nazareth is near Mount Carmel and Lake Galilee in Northern Israel, Bethlehem, Jerusalem and Qumran are in Southern Israel. Most of the events in Jesus life happened in Northern Israel. The feeding of the 5000, the Sermon on the Mount, the wedding at Cana, the calling of Andrew and Peter, the healing of the leper and many other events were in Northern Israel. John the Baptist was probably with the Qumran Essene community in southern Israel and is why he did not recognize Jesus when they met.

Mount Carmel was the headquarters of the entire Essene movement. In those days there was no town called "Nazareth" but it was a cooperative village of Essene Nazarenes. Jesus was referred to as a Nazarene which is a Northern Essene associated with Mount Carmel. In the book of ACTS, the early Christians are referred to as "the sect of the Nazarenes." They were not liked by the Jews in the Temple because they refused to sacrifice animals and were primarily vegetarians. That is why the New Testament states; "Nothing good can come from Nazareth (the Nazarenes.)"

The Catholic Bishop Epiphanius of Salamis on Cyprus from about 367 until 402, he was a monastic founder and was a witness to and participant in the troubled era after the Council of Nicaea. His book "*Panarion*," or "Medicine Chest," is an historical encyclopedia of ideas and movements and hotly contested topics in the fourth century. It treats about 77 religious sects and philosophies; detailing their histories, and rebutting their beliefs, it is an important historical document. It was written in *Koine* Greek and later translated into Latin, then English and other languages. His writings are found in Nag Hammadi and other Gnostic writings and in such patristic authors as Irenaeus, Hippolytus, and St. Augustine. Its translations have been found helpful to historians, church historians, students of Judasism and others interested in this time period.

In the book he admits that in his own day there still existed "Jewish Christians" called "Nazarenes" related to the ancient order of Essenes. Bishop Epiphanius admits also that the original followers of Jesus were "known as Nazarenes" and that "the sect of the Nazarenes existed prior to the birth of Jesus, they were of the descendant of the original Christianity. He denounced them because their beliefs differed from his as bishop. One of the things was that they were strict vegetarians. Thus in Bishop Epiphanius we have a fourth century witness of the original Christian sect of Nazarenes, directly connected to Jesus who was living as vegetarians. This is an extremely important document, it is evidence that is a historical statement in writing about this vegetarian community connected to and part of Jesus life from the fourth century, whom Jesus was part of and lived with as a vegetarian, according to them!

61. Question # Bib.61 Was James the Second Pope Kosher and Vegetarian?

One of the primary reasons that these Jewish people in community became vegetarian and upheld it was to fulfill the teachings of the Torah, God's Word. In Mosaic Law, blood must be strictly separated from food. (Lev 3:17; 7:26-27; 17:3-7; 10B14; 19:26; Deut 12:15-16, 20-28; 15:19-23; 1 Sam 14:32-35; Ex 33:25) The prohibition against eating blood was extremely important and even foreigners were not exempt (Lev 12:10-12). The easy way, in fact the only way to truly fulfill this requirement was to be vegetarian and not eat any meat that has blood in it.

James, a servant of God and of the Lord Jesus Christ (1.1), as the author of the *Epistle of James*, is not one of the twelve but the cousin of Jesus (Gal 1:19), and the administrator of the Jerusalem community (Ac 12:17). He played a leading role in the apostolic Council (Acts 15:13-21) forming the early Christian community. After Paul's third missionary journey they spoke in Jerusalem before Paul's arrest (Ac 21:17-25).

Peter was the first Bishop of the Church for a short time. After being rescued by the angel he had to flee the city. Then James took over as the head of the Jerusalem Church and of all that was first Christians. James, for two to three decades was the head of the early Church and in some ways the Bishop to both Peter and Paul. As the leader, James was clearly the undisputed successor to Jesus and certainly was 'the Bishop of Bishops' or 'Archbishop'. James is mentioned not only in the Gospels but also named or implied in other early writings from the Church Fathers, notably Origen, Eusebius, Epiphanisus, Hegesippus and Jerome. Also in some texts that are not accepted as part of the canon of Catholic Church books but historically they still have importance include: the *Gospel of Hebrews*, the *Gospel of Nazoraeans*, and the *Gospel of the Ebionites*, *Gnostic Gospel of Thomas*, the Pseudoclementine writings and the Apocryphal Gospel the *Protevangelium of James*. All this is important and James was an important figure in the very beginning of the Christian Church.

"According to the early Christian historian Hegesippus (2nd cent.), who is excerpted in Eusebius' *Ecclesiastical History*, 'James, the brother of the Lord, succeeded to the government of the Church in conjunction with the apostles. He has been called the Just by all from the time of our Savior to the present day for there were many called James. He was holy from his mother's womb and he drank no wine nor strong drink, nor did he eat flesh. No razor came upon his head; he did not anoint himself with oil, and he did not use the bath. He alone was permitted to enter into the holy place for he wore not woolen but linen garments...'"[80]

Yes, James the second Pope, "drank no wine nor strong drink, nor did he eat flesh" he was a vegetarian. He followed the kosher laws and Torah laws exactly which leads

a person to be a vegetarian. He also knew Jesus and Mary
and probably followed their example since they were model
vegetarians.

**62. Question # Bib.62   What did the Church Fathers
say about fasting and diet?**

Fasting is one of the cornerstones of the penitential
tradition. The Catholic Catechism mentions fasting as being
one of the five pillars of the Catholic Church. Looking at the
penitential practices in the first couple hundred years, a fast,
usually 6 to 7 days was a standard penance for wrong-doing;
or a practice that was done at Lent or other times. If most of
the billion Catholics did one or two 7 day fasts a year that
would save a lot of food to help the environment! Image if
all religions in the world fasted for 7 days once or twice a
year for themselves and world peace!

Fasting and food go together and were part of the
fabric of the biblical Jewish lifestyle. From scriptures to the
early Church Fathers fasting is part of the Christian way of
life. Clement of Alexandria (d. 202), making use of
scripture and philosophy, recommends frugality and
temperance to free oneself from matter.[81] For Origen,
fasting is an experience of freedom, not an obligation in view
of Pythagorean metapsychosis.[82] For Ambrose and Gregory
of Nyssa, mortification of the flesh puts man in communion
with Christ who raises him from human to a divine existence.[83]
For Basil, fasting guarantees peace in the world and in
families, because it frees people from egoism.[84] And for
Ambrose, it is the angelic life that leads us back to Paradise,
where 'sin entered through food'; 'those who do not believe
in the afterlife indulge in food and drink.'"[85]

"Monasticism carried the ascesis of fasting to
incredible heights. Anthony ate bread, water and salt.[86]
Pachomius fasted, but did not want his monks to lack food.[87]
For Jerome, the monk must always remain a little hungry: 'If

you wish to be perfect, it is better to fatten the soul than the body.'[88] Basil and Cassian recommended moderation, each one adapting the fast to his own situation.[89] St. Benedict's (d. 547) *Rule* recommends us to 'love fasting' with discretion.[90] While the monastic East explored the personal aspect, the Western communities looked to the social value. Leo the Great, who dedicated 30 treatises to fasting, said: 'the abstinence of him who fasts becomes the nourishment of the poor.'"[91]

St. Bernard in his Rule writes: "Renounce yourself in order to follow Christ (Mat 16:24; Lk 9:23); discipline your body (1 Cor 9:27); do not pamper yourself, but love fasting."[92] St. Francis of Assisi said, "All the friars without exception must fast ..."[93] St. Francis of Paola the miracle worker of Italy (1416 to 1507) also emphasized fasting in his rule.[94] Most founders of religious order required fasting.

The Divine Liturgy of St. Basil the Great (329-379) is still used in the Apostolic Eastern Traditions, both the Eastern rite and Byzantine tradition. St. Basil (4th century) the founder of monasticism, many of those in the early Church, and those in the first few hundred years of Christianity, emphasized fasting and a vegetarian diet.

The word "penance" has a history and going back to its roots it essentially means "purification" as found in Sacred Scripture. The penance or purification of the Church Fathers usually involved fasting, and, for serious sins, people would be given the penance of fasting for a whole week in the early Church. Fasting was not just for sins but for emotional distress, as with David who fasted for six days at the death of someone, or for other spiritual activities.

Modern day fasting is considered a purification of the body since dead, diseased and dying cells are flushed out of the system during a fast. Fasting detoxifies a person and it also rebalance a person's biochemistry. Fasting therapy is usually two to three weeks or longer, it is very successfully being used for degenerative diseases and illnesses. Fasting has healed hundreds of thousands of people and before the advent of pharmaceutical drugs, fasting was a primary means of curing people of diseases.[95]

As Christians, fasting is part of our life, it is not an option. If Moses, who beheld God, (on Sinai) and St. Paul, the divine apostle (Act 9:9) fasted, so must we. If the Ninevites fasted (Jonah 3:5), and this included all their children plus their 'senior' citizens, so we must. If the Church Fathers and the Saints expect us to fast, so, must we. Finally, if Jesus Himself fasted and was hungry (Lk 4:2), who are we to introduce a 'new improved and fast-free' spirituality?

Jesus gave an admonition telling people to fast: "Moreover, when you fast..." Mt 6:16 At the death of Saul, "they fasted for seven days." 1 Ch 10:12, 1 Sam 31:13. Many more examples can be given of fasting in the Bible. David's lament humbled himself with fasting; Ps 102.4, "Yet, when they were sick, I put sackcloth on, I humbled my soul with fasting." Ps 35:13 "On a fast day...you shall read the words of the Lord." Jer 36.6

Fasting has been healing people since Biblical times. Today there are fasting centers that have helped cure major illness and degenerative diseases.[96] A list of healings can be given for those on a vegetarian, strict vegan, and raw vegan diet, often referred to as Living Foods. These strict raw vegan diets can put into remission or cure all kinds of diseases like cancer, MS and Parkinson's.[97] Healing, fasting and a penitential diet (i.e. vegetarian, vegan, raw vegan) are part of the fabric of the Christian Church.

Healing indeed plays a large role in the Gospel, where four different verbs are used to express it. The third is *katharizo*, which means "purify"[e] (Mt 8:2,3; 11:5; Mk 1:40;

_____

[e] (Mt 8:2,3; 11:5; Mk 1:40; Lk 5:12; 17:14)

Lk 5:12; 17:14). This is a very significant insight since back in Biblical times for a person to be cured meant that they were purified or cleansed. And the concept of eating a Kosher diet or fasting is for the sake of purification.

A Fatima scholar Fr. Antonio Martins, SJ explains how sin yields punishment, "According to the Bible, there is an intrinsic co-relation between sin and affliction, between obedience to God and happiness. The Hebrew Scriptures point out how sin yields punishment. This is also found in some verses in the New Testament, … But men prefer to be slaves of their own degrading and unruly passions."[98] Starting out in the book of Judges and Deuteronomy, (Jg. 2:11-15; Dt. 11:26-28) we pass to I and II Samuel, we find the same thesis of sin followed inexorably by chastisement. If from the historical books we pass on to the prophets, we can verify that the idea of sin being followed by punishment is emphasized with even greater vigor. It suffices to read Hosea 13:1-15; Amos 2:1-16; 3:11; 6:6-9; Micah 3:1-12, in order to be completely convinced. Some will obviously disagree but, "There is a way that some think right, but it leads in the end to death." (Prov. 14:12).[99]

This "sin yields punishment" could apply on the personal level of health involving the activities of our flesh and degenerative diseases. It also involves the corporate level of a city or a country or the world in this topic of climate change: Global warming and Global depletion.

The time has come he said and the kingdom of God is close at hand. Reform or purify your lives and believe the Good News. Mk 1:15 "Jesus Christ required purification and remission of sins should be preached to all nations." Lk 24.47 "Watch and pray, that ye enter not into temptation." Mt 26:41

Notice:
If this book is a significant help to your health or illness or degenerative disease, or even beneficial or a conversion or faith walk, please let us know. Myself and my associates are collecting testimonials and case studies for future works and possible a book. We are always interested when this book helps you in you're: body, soul or spirit. Drop us a letter. I do not always reply to email, but I always reply to a snail mail, drop me a letter or communicate.

For other related books or activities see the website: www.jimtibbetts.com   Thank you and God bless.

Sincerely in Christ

Jim Tibbetts

63. Appendix

A. Bio - James C. Tibbetts

Jim Tibbetts has an MBA (2009); an STL (1995) in Marian Studies (International Marian Research Institute, Univ. Dayton, Ohio) and an MA (1983) in theology (Univ. Steubenville, Ohio). He is a member of Secular Franciscan Order, the K of C and the American Mariological Society. James as a businessman ran various businesses and has worked with the mentally handicapped. As a theologian he has given talks at national conferences, society meetings and given retreats on; Spirituality, Marian topics; on plant-based diets, fasting, healing and Christian meditation. He has been into a plant-based diet and seven day juice fasting since late 1970's and has done over 40 long juice fasts.

Jim produced several DVD's on spiritual topics and mime. From 1978 to 2003, Jim was a professional mime; solo, duet and was a founding member (1991 to 2001) of the group "Christsong" which performed around the U.S., twice-toured England and appeared on television shows. "Tibbetts has studied his art under technique-oriented Marcel Marceau and personality-oriented Tony Montanaro. The result has been a critically acclaimed combination of the two." (*Arts & Entertainment*, Evening Express, Portland, ME.)

Jim developed and leads the Rosary Yoga (and Pilates) with groups, a posture for each bead and he promotes Christian Yoga. He has written journal and popular articles and has written over 20 books including:

1. Juice Fasting Simplified, a Practical Approach
2. A Diary on Juice Fasting
3. Living Green with Juices, Smoothies and Salads with Anne Marie Tibbetts, MS, RD
4. Starving Cancer to Death, Nutritional Integrative Cancer Therapies, with Joseph Spaziani, MD
5. Starving into Remission: Alzheimer's, Parkinson's

and Multiple Sclerosis - Nutritional Therapies
with Anne Marie Tibbetts, MS, RD

6. The Bioethics of Drug Intervention
7. Superior Health for Astronauts as Raw Vegans
   A Nutrition Novel
8. Christian Meditation, the Jesus Prayer and Praise
9. Jesus and Mary were Kosher Vegetarian, the Evidence
   from the Bible, the Early Church and Nutrition (2014)
10. Biblical Nutrition and Fasting (2008)
11. Biblical Nutrition; Forty Days of Meditations (2004)
12. Biblical Nutrition the Kosher Vegetarianism
    of Jesus and Judaism (2003)
13. Biblical Fasting (1998)
14. A Biblical Ballad of Mary Mother of Jesus
15. Biblical Titles of the Virgin Mary - 30 Day Meditation
16. Mary the Kosher Vegetarian, Impacting Climate Change
17. Mary the Ark of the Covenant with Fr. Bill McCarthy
18. Guadalupe the Tilma's Conquest - a historical novel
19. Q&A about Vegetarians and Health

Jim Tibbetts
P.O. Box 2533
Glenville, NY 12325
www.jimtibbetts.com

64. Endnotes

[1] Kalechofsky, Roberta, *Judaism and Animal Rights*, (Micah Pub. Marblehead, MA., 2002) Rabbi Noach Valley, p. 201.

[2] Schwartz, Richard, Ph.D., *Vegetarianism and the Jewish Dietary Laws*, p. 4, The Schwartz Collection... (on his website).

[3] (Lev 10:10; 11:47; 20:25; Ezek 22:26)

[4] cleanness (Lev 15:13; 22:4); to cleanse (Lev 16:30; Num 8:6); to cleanse oneself (Num 8:7; Josh 22:17); purifying (Lev 12:4); cleansing (Lev 13:7: Num 6:9); clean (Gen 7:2; Lev 11:47)

[5] (Lev 14:52; Num 19:19; Ezek 43:20), and to cleanse oneself (Num 19:12-13, 20).

[6] (Job 15:14; 25:4; 33:9; Ps 73;13; Isa 1:16)

[7] (Is 35:8; 52:1; Ezek 39:24; Rev 21:27), or is... opposed to God (Zech 13:2; Mk 1:23; Lk 4:33; Ac 5:16), and ...abomination to Yahweh (Lev 7:21; 11:10; Deut 17:1).

[8] Schwartz, *Judaism and Vegetarianism*, p. 121, citing: Rabbi J. David Bleich, "Vegetarianism and Judaism," *Tradition*, Vol. 23, No. 1 (summer, 1987).

[9] Dionysius the Areopagite, *The Divine Names and Mystical Theology*, trans by C.E. Rolt, (SPCK, Holy Trinity Church, London, 1979), p. 55.

[10] Russell, Rex, M.D., *What the Bible Says About Healthy Living*, on the page 150. David Macht, M.D., "An Experimental Pharmacological Appreciation of Leviticus XI and Deuteronomy XIV," *Bulletin of Historical Medicine*, Johns Hopkins University, 47:1 (April 1953): pp. 444-450.

[11] Russell, Rex, M.D., *What the Bible Says About Healthy Living*, p. 150. Citing: David Macht, M.D., "An Experimental Pharmacological Appreciation of Leviticus XI and Deuteronomy XIV," *Bulletin of Historical Medicine*, Johns Hopkins University, 47:1 (April 1953): pp. 444-450.

[12] Russell, Rex, M.D., *What the Bible Says About Healthy Living*, p. 150. Citing: David Macht, M.D., "An Experimental Pharmacological Appreciation of Leviticus XI and Deuteronomy XIV," *Bulletin of Historical Medicine*, Johns Hopkins University, 47:1 (April 1953): pp. 444-450.

[13] Ehret, Arnold, *Rational Fasting*, (Benedict Lust Publications, New York, NY, 1917), also, Beneficial Books, 1977, p. 67, 49.

[14] Russell, Rex, M.D., *What the Bible Says About Healthy Living*, (Regal Books, Ventura, CA., 1996), p. 43. Citing: M.A. Ruffer, "Studies in Paleopathology in Egypt," *Journal of Pathology and Bacteriology* 18 (1913): 149-62; P.E. Ross, "Eloquent Remains," *Scientific American* 266:5 (May 1992): 114-19; C.T. Marx, "Examination of Eleven Egyptian Mummies," *RasioGraphics* 6:2 (March 1986): 321-325.

[15] Russell, Rex, *What the Bible Says...* p. 43.
[16] From the Institute of Judeo-Christian Studies at Seton Hall University, South Orange, NJ 07079.
[17] Lawrence E. Frizzell, *Marian Studies*, XLVI (University of Dayton, Ohio, 1995), p. 27; citing: See John M. Oesterreicher, "Piety and Prayer in the Jewish Home," *Worship* 27(1953): 540-549.
[18] See Mary Douglas in an appendix to Jacob Neusner, *The Idea of Purity in Judaism* (Leiden: E.J. Brill, 1973, 137-142. The diagram, which is based on her work, is my own (Frizzell).
[19] Lawrence E. Frizzell, *Marian Studies*, XLVI (1995), p. 32.
[20] "Our Lady of Eden 1974 *Marian Studies* Marian Library, University of Dayton, Ohio.
[21] Citing: St. Jerome, St. Augustine, St. Cyril of Jerusalem, St. John Chryostom, St. John Damascene. This is stated in the *Documents of Vatican II* (LG 56); and in the *Catechism of the Catholic Church* (494).
[22] Buby, Bertrand, SM, *Mary of Galilee, The Marian Heritage of the Early Church*, Alba House, New York, NY, 1995, (New York: Scribner=s, 1926), 249. citing: Irenaeus *Against Heresies*, XXII, 4; Roberts and Donaldson, op. cit., vol. 1, 449, p. 20.
[23] See Jim Tibbetts books (Charlton, NY) as previously noted..
[24] Kalchofsky, Roberta, *Vegetarian Judaism*, (Micah Publications, Inc., N.H. 1998), p. 168.
[25] Stegemann, Hartmut, *The Library of Qumran, On the Essenes, Qumran, John the Baptist, and Jesus* (William B. Eerdman's Publishing Company, Grand Rapids, Michigan, (1993 German) 1998 English), 267.
[26] *Encyclopedia of the Dead Sea Scrolls*, Editors Schiffman, VanderKam, p. 813, citing: *Jewish Antiquities* 13.171-173.
[27] *Encyclopedia of the Dead Sea...*, p. 264, citing: *The Jewish War* 2.145.
[28] *Encyclopedia of the Dead Sea...*, p. 264, citing: *The Jewish War* 2.136.
[29] *Encyclopedia of the Dead Sea Scrolls*, p. 264, citing: *Refutatio* 9.27.
[30] *Encyclopedia of the Dead Sea Scrolls*, p. 266, citing: 1 QS iv.6-8; CD iii.20; see also *Rule of Blessings* (1Q28b) iv.24-26.
[31] *Encyclopedia of the Dead Sea Scrolls*, p. 266, citing: 4Q521.
[32] Kalechofsky, *Vegetarian Judaism*, (Micah Publications, Inc., N.H. 1998), p. 48.
[33] Feeley-Harnik, Gillian, Smithsonian Institution Press, Washington, D.C., 1994, p. 105, citing: *Flaccus*, 95-6.
[34] Feeley-Harnik, Gillian, p. 106, citing: *The Jewish War*, 2:152-53.
[35] Ewing, Upton Clary, *The Prophet of the Dead Sea Scrolls* (Tree of Life Publications, Joshua Tree, CA, 1993; 1963), p. 85, citing: Josephus *Life*, 3.
[36] Ewing, Upton Clary, Tree of Life Publications, Joshua Tree, CA, 1993 (1963), p. 85, citing: Josephus *Life*, 3.
[37] Thiering, Barbara, "The Biblical Source of Qumran Asceticism", p. 431, University of Sydney, Sydney, Australia, *Journal of Biblica Literature* Thiering, vol. 93, 1974, pp. 429-444.

[38] Thiering, Barbara, "The Biblical Source of Qumran Asceticism", p. 443, citing: *Ant.* 13.11,1; 311; 15.105; 337; 17.5,6; 346.

[39] Cousens, Gabriel, MD, *Creating Peace by Being Peace, p. 6.*

[40] Ewing, *The Prophet of the Dead Sea Scrolls*, p. 122-123.

[41] Ewing, *The Prophet of the Dead Sea Scrolls*, p. 122-123.

[42] Rabbi Gabriel Cousens, *Modern Essenes A Brief Synopsis*, a handout (Monday July 2, 2012) at the Tree of Life conference for the Essene Gathering.

[43] Pope Benedict XVI (Joseph Ratzinger), *Jesus of Nazareth, Holy Week: From the Entrance into Jerusalem to the Resurrection*, (Ignatius Press, San Francisco, 2011, Hardbound edition Doubleday Publishing), p. 106, 110, 111.

[44] Pope Benedict XVI, *Jesus of Nazareth*, p. 224-225, citing: the French exegete Henri Cazelles, drawing on studies by J. Collson, J. Winandy, and M.E. Boismard. Cazelles, *"Johannes"* p. 481, pp. 480, 481.

[45] Rabbi Gabriel Cousens, *Modern Essenes, A Brief Synopsis*, a handout (Monday July 2, 2012) at the Tree of Life conference for the Essene Gathering.

[46] Rabbi Gabriel Cousens, *Modern Essenes, A Brief Synopsis*, a handout (Monday July 2, 2012) at the Tree of Life conference for the Essene Gathering.

[47] Joseph Cardinal Ratzinger released a document (Rome, the feast of the Ascension 2001) by the Pontifical Biblical Commission: *The Jewish People and Their Sacred Scriptures in the Christian Bible*, it speaks several times of the Essenes.

[48] Joseph Cardinal Ratzinger released a document (Rome, the feast of the Ascension 2001) by the Pontifical Biblical Commission: *The Jewish People and Their Sacred Scriptures in the Christian Bible*, it speaks several times of the Essenes.

[49] Pope Benedict XVI (Joseph Ratzinger) *Jesus of Nazareth, from the Baptism in the Jordan to the Transfiguration*, (Ignatius Press, San Francisco, 2007, Hardbound edition Doubleday Publishing).

[50] Pope Benedict XVI, *Jesus of Nazareth,* p. 13, 14.

[51] Brown, Raphael, *The Life of Mary as Seen by the Mystics*, Tan Books and Publishers, Rockford, IL, 1951, reprinted 1991).

[52] Brown, Raphael, *The Life of Mary as Seen by the Mystics*, p. 96.

[53] Pope Benedict XVI (Joseph Ratzinger) *Jesus of Nazareth, from the Baptism in the Jordan to the Transfiguration*, (Ignatius Press, San Francisco, 2007, Hardbound edition Doubleday Publishing).

[54] Pope Benedict XVI, *Jesus of Nazareth,* p. 13, 14.

[55] McGowan, *Ascetic Eucharist's, Food and Drink,* (Clarendon Press Oxford, New York, 1999), p. 78, citing: Philo, *Prob.* 72-91; *Hypoth.* 11:1-18; *Cont.* 1-90.

[56] McGowan, *Ascetic Eucharists,* p. 78 citing: Josephus, *Jewish Wars* 1:3:78-80; 2:7:111-13; 2:8:119-61; 2:20:566-8. Antiquities 13:59:171-2; 18:15:18-22.

[57] McGowan, *Ascetic Eucharists,* p. 78 citing: Pliny the Elder, *Natural History* 5:17:4.

[58] Ibid., described in 1QS 6:4-5; 1QSa 2:11-22

[59] McGowan, *Ascetic Eucharists,* p. 78 citing: K.H. Kuhn, "The Lord's Supper and the communal meal at Qumran", in K. Stendahl (ed.), *The Scrolls and the New Testament,* 1958, pp. 65-93; J. van der Ploeg, "The meals of the Essenes", JSS 2, 1957, pp. 163-75; E.F. Sutcliffe, "Sacred meals at Qumran?", *Heythrop Journal* 1, 1960, pp. 48-65.

[60] Kalechofsky, *Judaism and Animal Rights,* p. 150-51, citing: Louis A. Berman, *The Dietary Laws as Atonements for Flesh-eating.*

[61] Kalechofsky, *Judaism and Animal..,* p. 151, citing: Baba Batra 60b.

[62] See Jewish Vegetarian Society or Professor Kalechofsky, PhD writings on Jewish vegetarianism.

[63] *Encyclopedia of the Early Church,* Institutum Patristicum Augustinianum, (Oxford University Press, Inc., New York, N.Y., 1992).

[64] *Encyclopedia of the Early Church,* citing: Iren., *Haer.* I 2,1 ; Tertull., *Ieiun.* 15, 1; Epiph., *Haer.* 30,18ff. and 47,1; Aug., *Haer.* 25.46.70.

[65] Ewing, *The Prophet of the Dead Sea Scrolls,* p. 145, citing: *Hastings Encyclopedia on Religion and Ethics* (V.5, p. 143), Charles Scribner's, Sons, N.Y.

[66] Ewing, *The Prophet of the Dead Sea Scrolls,* p. 145, citing: Teicher, J.L., *Journal of Jewish Studies,* 1951.

[67] As explained in *A Critical Investigation of Epiphanius' Knowledge of the Ebionites: A Translation and Critical Discussion of "Panarion,"* by Glen Alan Kochit.

[68] Cousens, Gabriel, *Conscious Eating,* p. 381.

[69] *Encyclopedia of the Dead Sea Scrolls,* Editors Schiffman, VanderKam, p. 248, citing: *Adversus omnes Haereses* 1.28.

[70] *Encyclopedia of the Early Church,* Institutum Patristicum Augustinianum, Oxford University Press, Inc., New York, N.Y., 1992.

[71] *Encyclopedia of the Early Church,* citing: Hermas, *Past., Sim.* V 1,5; cf. Emped. fr B144.

[72] *Encyclopedia of the Early Church,* citing: *ibid.* V3, 7; cf. Cypr., *Or* 32-33

[73] *Encyclopedia of the Early Church,* citing: Hermas, *Past., Sim* 3,9.

[74] *Encyclopedia of the Early Church,* citing: Clem. Al., *Paed.* II, 1, 1 ff.; Tertull., *Cult. fem* II 9.7; Orig., *In Jer.* 20,7; Euseb., *HE* V 3,2 and d.e.3, 5; Jerome, Jov. 5,18.

[75] *Encyclopedia of the Early Church,* citing: Can. ap. 50 and 52.

[76] *Encyclopedia of the Early Church,* citing: Iren., *Haer.* I 2,1 ; Tertull., *Ieiun.* 15, 1; Epiph., *Haer.* 30,18ff. and 47,1; Aug., *Haer.* 25.46.70.

[77] *Encyclopedia of the Early Church,* citing: *Ps Clem. rec.* VII 6,4; cf. Greg. Naz., *Or.* 14,4.

[78] Grimm, Veronika, E., *From Feasting to Fasting, the Evolution of Sin, Attitudes to food in late Antiquity,* New York, NY: Routledge, 1996. p. 97-98.

[79] Grimm, *From Feasting to Fasting, the Evolution of Sin*, p. 105, 106, citing: *Stromateis* 2:20.

[80] McGowan, Andrew, *Ascetic Eucharists, Food and Drink in Early Christian Ritual Meals*, (Clarendon Press Oxford, New York, 1999), p. 149.

[81] *Encyclopedia of the Early Church*, (Institutum Patristicum Augustinianum, Oxford University Press, New York, N.Y., 1992), citing: Paed. II 1, 1-2, 34; III 12, 90.

[82] *Encyclopedia of the Early Church*, citing: Cels. 5, 49 and 8, 30.

[83] *Encyclopedia of the Early Church*, citing: In *Lev.* 10, 1-2; cf. Ambr., *In Ps.* 40, 1: Greg. Nyss., Beat. IV; Util. ieiun. 1,1.

[84] *Encyclopedia of the Early Church*, citing: Basil, Ieiun. Hom. 2, 5; cf. Chrom., Serm. 35.4 and In Mt. 29.

[85] *Encyclopedia of the Early Church*, citing: Ambr., Hel. 3,4; 4,7; Ep 63, 17).

[86] *Encyclopedia of the Early Church*, citing: Athan., Ant. 7,6.

[87] *Encyclopedia of the Early Church*, citing: Via Pach. 25.

[88] *Encyclopedia of the Early Church*, citing: Jov. 2,6; Ep 54, 105.

[89] *Encyclopedia of the Early Church*, citing: Basil, *Ieiun.* 1 and 2; Cass., *Coll* 21.13ff, and Inst. *coen.* 5,5 ff; cf. Hipp., *Trad.* ap. 25; Epiph., *Haer.* 3; Exp. *fid.* 23; Theodor., *Haer. fab.* 5,29.

[90] *Encyclopedia of the Early Church*, citing: Rule 4,39-41, 49.

[91] *Encyclopedia of the Early Church*, citing: 12-20; 39-50; 86-94, *Serm.* 13,1.

[92] *St. Benedict's Rule for Monasteries*, (Liturgical Press, Collegeville, Minnesota, 1948), citing Chapter 1, p. 6.

[93] *St. Francis of Assisi, Omnibus of Sources*, (Franciscan Herald Press, Chicago, Illinois, 1983), p. 34.

[94] Vanzillotta, Gino, O.M., books: *The Third Order of Minims* (Los Angeles, CA., 2001); *Francis the "Minim"* (Los Angeles, CA., 2001); *Life of St. Francis of Paola*, translation, written by: Anonymous Disciple Contemporary with the Saint (Los Angeles, CA., 2002).

[95] James and Anne Marie Tibbetts, *Juice Fasting a Practical Approach* (Glenville, NY, 2008).

[96] See Jim Tibbetts book on *Juice Fasting* or Dr. Herbert M. Shelton's book *Fasting for the Health* of it with their examples of cures.

[97] James Tibbetts, Joseph Spaziani, *Starving Cancer to Death* (2007); James Tibbetts, Anne Marie Tibbetts, Remission towards Curing: Alzheimer's, Parkinson's and Multiple Sclerosis Nutritional Integrative Therapies (2014).

[98] Martins, Antonio, S.J., *Fatima Way of Peace*, (Still River, MA., The Ravengate Press, 1989), p. 23-24.

[99] Martins, Antonio, S.J., *Fatima Way of Peace*, (Still River, MA., The Ravengate Press, 1989), p. 23-24.

Notes

www.ingramcontent.com/pod-product-compliance
Lightning Source LLC
Chambersburg PA
CBHW052246290526
45785CB00016B/1402